DEA
STREETS

Shane Leah

chipmunkapublishing
the mental health publisher
empowering people with schizophrenia

30127074386959

Shane Leah

Published by
Chipmunkapublishing
PO Box 6872
Brentwood
Essex CM13 1ZT
United Kingdom

http://www.chipmunkapublishing.com

Chipmunkapublishing gratefully acknowledge the support of Arts Council England.

Suffolk County Council	
07438695	
Askews	Jul-2009
	£10.00

DEAD CITY STREETS

Preface

Fear: my initial purpose and reason for living the life I have the way I do, was, and still is, to find a life partner I love. Unfortunately, the sum of my teens became evident in my twenties, when I was diagnosed with a mental illness. The result being that the first word of this paragraph is what has become of those innocent aspirations to fall in love; that is, I have crippling doubts.

The reason as I understand it is that my formative teenage years, when I was at college, were not an entirely happy time in my life.

You see, some time after my 13th birthday in the April of 1993, I was introduced to the scourge of my life, Cannabis. Now, in all honesty I still smoke and often enjoy doing so, but I realise now that its effect on my life has been to limit my plans and goals, to the point where I am losing out to the competition. But this is in effect the symptom, not the cause.

'I have been disappointed in love.' Should I die today then this is what I want as my epitaph, simply because I am tired of making excuses for my emotional choices, and this I feel, is the real reason for my sickness after the millennium period when I suffered a breakdown I have since recovered from.

The problem is I was often criticised by some members of my social circle for my melancholic feelings and inertia when it came to capitalising upon sexual advances that I would have sooner investigated before committing myself to their cause.

All I can say in my defence is that we are not alike. Back when I was 19, I did love my girlfriend as much as anything I have ever had as my own.

So to be true, I know now that the reason for my unhappy late teens and schizophrenic twenties, is that every suggestion of doubt planted in my mind by those who were not as confident about my relationship as I was back then, finally resulted in me succumbing to the worldly way of doing things devoid of emotion.

To conclude, the reason for my breakdown and illness that lasted many years is simply these seeds of doubt have become my worries, anxieties, and fears. This is the root cause of my illness.

DEAD CITY STREETS

Chapter 1

Losing Something

My early childhood was a happy one. I had two wonderful parents who loved me and my two brothers and sister (later to become two) dearly and we grew up in relative comfort and safety in a more stable environment than you would of expected. I certainly had no real reason to follow the path I set out upon as a teenager. I did however have an excuse. My parents separated when I was eight, later getting divorced about a year later and I have to say it was a selfish decision, as the marriage was probably worth saving... Regardless of this they maintained their commitment to us children and they continue to love us to this day. In all honesty I cannot criticise them for their decision, as it gave us children more freedom than we could have ever used - maybe too much in my case, as events would transpire.

I was never witness or victim of any kind of abuse as a young child, be it serious or just domestic. Our family and those of the neighbours around the housing estate we lived on were average and stable, though the teenagers often rebelled against their teachings and better learning by using drink and drugs and becoming involved in petty crime. The group of friends I belonged to all of the same age group often followed them around or watched their movements in an effort to learn what it meant to be an adult. In hindsight I can see each generation is pretty much the same between the ages of thirteen to twenty five, when they have to learn the laws of society while pushing the boundaries of how much fun they can have. I should have watched and learned more. I suppose I had no recognition of the dangers of the world at that age, though the lessons I was to learn myself were all there around me if I had just opened my eyes and took note of the actions of those teenagers I knew.

We moved house in the winter of '91, to another street not far away to escape the trouble brewing on the estate we lived as families began falling apart through death or divorce and their children began expressing their anger and frustration. Their powerlessness to control their security and happiness resulted in small scale confrontations with the police and an explosion of drug abuse and misuse on the streets of home. Even television report actively encouraged the challenging authority and the individual rights of the new generation, who wanted an alternative to the home and family which had failed them. Drugs and music seemed the answer. Thus the nineties were bore out of this 'hash' of young ideas and the inability of the society we lived in to hold itself together cohesively within the myths of the older generation. That is love, career, home and family. All of which you must be privileged to be part of in my generation. We needn't of bothered running, it caught up with me and my older brother soon enough.

Our new home was in a part of town occupied by large families of four children or more. Some had

DEAD CITY STREETS

as many as twelve and though poverty was an issue, neglect was even more prevalent; but we settled in and began making a new life for ourselves. My mother made some new friends and so did we; my siblings and I. Soon I was dating girls and staying out late with my older brother, smoking and drinking cheap beer. The good times rolled on for about a year as we experimented with sex and drink and cigarettes. I became interested in music and started playing guitar on a Friday at a neighbour's house and I progressed onto vodka - these were the good times. But soon I was to experiment with the dirge of my life and the one thing I could have avoided and saved myself the trouble of being abused at the hands of my supply, Cannabis. Thing is, having started I never looked back until I was twenty five and only by then could I see what effect it had on my life.

My first experience of drugs was a shady one that I soon got used to. We (my friends and I), were riding a 'borrowed' motorcycle round an old abandoned road near some wasteland known as 'Jacks Wood,' when a young homeless boy of about eighteen approached us from some bushes and threatened to 'mess up' one of my friends. My friends knew him it seemed as someone with mental problems as he was positively schizophrenic in his attitude towards us first threatening us then asking how we were and what we were up to, before turning on us again and attempting to steal our motorcycle.

My friend retaliated by making threats to tell *the*

madman's father where the guy was, and what he was doing there camping out in the wood. A tat for tat commotion ensued and we started walking away leaving the bike behind for him to take. He then attempted to set fire to it and then walked away himself. Seeing our chance to retrieve it one of us raced back to pick it up and we set off home. But not before he stopped at the end of the road, just before he was to disappear into the wood and shouted back, 'Anyone want to buy any weed?' I wasn't the only one to hesitate and stop. One of my friends asked, in nervous anxiety more than anything if any of us wanted any. I made a stupid, nervous decision myself and took a five pound note I had earned that morning, delivering milk from my new wallet and offered it to my friend who had queried our desire to become junkies. He didn't take it and instead suggested that I go back and buy the shit. Which I did, and returned with some of the finest quality 'Lebanese' hashish I have ever smoked. That's pollen to you and me…

Around the corner from the wood I considered what I had just bought. My friends and I were excited due to the encounter and the result, and questions came from all directions about my intent. Was I going to smoke it and end up like him - the guy in the wood? Or should I throw it away…the choice was mine but the pressure was now definitely on. Struggling with what I had been taught about drugs and the disappointment of wasting a fiver, it took several minutes, to the far side of the footbridge over the railway to make my decision. I thought what my father would say and threw it on the floor in the alley amongst all the dog dirt and chip wrappers.

You would have thought that would be the last of the story. Unfortunately for my mental health, it was not.

After that day I would go on to smoke heavily till I was 15, when I stopped to concentrate on my GCSE exams. I then continued to smoke once I reached 6th form, only heavier. Soon I became involved in a seedy underworld of speed and teenage single mothers. I was never sure I really liked my new delinquent friends, as I had noble and laudable dreams of becoming a doctor of child psychology!

Anyway the story goes that before long I was introduced to a friend of a friend who had just been released from prison and became his confidant. He shall go unnamed as such, but in the years that followed I was very much his right hand man and my feelings for the man were strong. I was genuinely loyal to him and his young partner and family; that I hasten to add he seemed ashamed of? Unfortunately the 'steep' was slippery and in the light of his past conviction and my naivety by 18, I was embroiled in the depressing world of cocaine and domestic abuse. I really was very unhappy.

And so in the time between the millennium celebrations and September of the New Year, I became so embittered by the constant fights between the three of us in our téte á téte - plus one, that I finally left home to take my life.

Miss 8 years therapy and you have me here today by the grace of the NHS staff, who have supported me throughout my 'illness'. I am eternally grateful for the support I gained despite the trial and retribution I have suffered. It would appear I am not responsible for my actions...

And guess who that friend was back then? I feel sorry for the future I may have had...

DEAD CITY STREETS

Chapter 2

Wirral Gig

The night when I first had been alone, I was one of only two passengers on the last train west from my home town. Problems at home had been causing me a lot of distress. I hated the tiny box room I had to sleep in at night, allocated to me after I moved back to my mothers from my digs I had shared with a friend. My flatmate had evicted me after I smashed up the house on a narced out rage. I had also acquired some huge debts as a result of getting involved with drugs, specifically speed when I was away from home. Me and my mother weren't getting on very well and all my support networks that made my life what it was had collapsed upon leaving work. Even my brothers were ill at ease with me. Worse of all I was twenty and alone after splitting from my girlfriend.

Of course I had become quite insane during this time as I had a lot of emotional pain going on in my life and though it wasn't uncommon for me to like a drink and a smoke, my mind had been so mashed during my benders alone at home that I made little sense to those around me and who consequentially had become worried about my behaviour. I experienced audible hallucinations, and would talk at length with the disembodied voices of my parents and friends and figures long gone from my life. I also began to express some strange, I might add false beliefs that worried everyone including myself. This was the onset of my illness.

As it progressed I became disorientated and isolated from my family and friends who could not understand my behaviour. I became a stranger in my own household, distant and removed from those people I loved. Filled with hate and rage I began pressing my distress upon my friends. But none could understand my questions, let alone tell me what I wanted to hear. Soon they had fallen out with me too and having no one I could hang out with, I began to wander round the streets at night with my dog, not knowing what it was I was looking for. Love was my quandary. And as God spoke to me I looked inward to find the satisfaction I sought. The one I loved and craved was far away.

What makes the story complete though is the events of the day I left my mother with thoughts of horror as I crazily drove a pile through the relationships in my life by leaving my girl alone in the hands of a friend with little respect for me. The story I am about to tell is the secret history of the love affair in the decadent turn of the century and the concerns of a broken home. Its legacy mental illness.

My mother was getting ready for a blazing night out on the tiles with her friend from the south, Bette. So were her two youngest children, Gareth and Nardia, who were making preparations to spend the night at a friends' across town. As they rushed about running baths and ironing clothes, they did not notice the behaviour of they're Brother Shane, who had been feeling uncomfortable for some time. He was not eating properly and he had become a devil to deal with. They were not going to let him ruin they're night tonight. He loitered about the place, not resting anywhere and complaining he had nowhere to go and felt lonely this Christmas Eve. They took this attitude as a machination to prevent them from having any fun, which they had been having plenty of since he moved out. But now he had returned after losing his job at the cement works and having been made homeless he had moved back to the family home. Sick of his sulking Annette suggested him go and see one of his friends Sim, but he knew he wasn't welcome. It was a family Christmas, and that he wasn't. She phoned another of his friends Howie, and made arrangements for him to go round but instead of accepting the invitation he complained he was bored of they're company and would sooner stay in. She could take no more of his attitude and demanded that he was not at home when she returned, as she would have company. As the partygoers all left home one by one, to go to their destinations, he sat alone upstairs in the junk room feeling sorry for himself. The weed he had smoked earlier began to take hold of his mind and as the clock struck just before midnight he slipped out of the house and into the darkness of night taking his dog Faith, with him.

I left my home one cold night at Christmas Eve before the millennium. With my giro money in my pocket I was going to take the train to Hooton, but upon encountering the memory of an *old ghost* on the opposite seat I took the chance to get off at the next stop, Eastham Rake. Taking my dog with me I walked along the lanes to the next town, stopping at the grammar school to make a joint and then on to the countryside through the fields. Gazing at the stars and the waxing full moon I wondered if there was something up there that could help me in my search to find some comfort. A hot meal, a comfortable bed, the love of a family any would bring me the joy I needed. But none were to be found out here. I was an outsider a vagrant even, and I was. The millennium held no new start for me. The situation at home had been bad enough to drive me away but out here I was at the mercy of the elements. There was little hope for me getting back on my feet again. By now the weed was causing ruptures in my thinking and I kept walking not knowing my destination.

As I traveled the roads became more winding and the rain drenched the tarmac and the plains around me. Each time a car approached I had to throw myself into the bushes, as I was dressed in black (as was my dog) and the drivers could not see us at the side of the road. Each of them missed us by centimeters nearly taking us both out. I made progress through the night slowly, not even knowing where I was.

Turning 'this way and that' I searched for direction letting the landscape and the smell and sound of the night air influence me on my course. By now I was very tired and I focused on my energy on finding somewhere to sleep and so continued walking, looking for a barn or shed in which to doss for the night. As I entered the village of Storeton, I kept my eyes peeled for a suitable resting place. But it seemed all eyes were on me here. I walked to the green then doubled back on myself and took a right down a bridal path and into the fields beyond. Ahead of me was a hay barn down a dirt track next to a farmhouse. I decided to stop here. I made my way towards it with my dog limping beside me. I had walked twenty miles or more into the night and now needed to rest. The barn was draught-proof between the huge round bales of hay stacked high above me. I found an enclosure between some bales and settled down for the remainder of the morning. As the suns rays breached the horizon and the rain clouds gathered, I settled into my slumber and drifted off to sleep as the dog wandered around the farmyard.

The O'Malley's woke Christmas day to the sun blazing through the crystal blue clear skies above the fields to the south of the farm and rain clouds gathering in the east. The children sat at their table in the kitchen and waited for their Christmas fry up. Outside the dogs were let out into the yard from their kennels and immediately sensed an intruder. Jack O'Malley hesitated, thinking someone had taken some piece of equipment in the night and put his Wellingtons on and ventured out to see. Past the gate to the livestock barn he could see the cattle had been startled and would not be giving milk. Angry, he went back to the house to fetch his air-gun and then ventured round the yard looking to take a shot. A lone Labrador stood in the yard shaking its tail. Someone was here. He had just closed the gate when a husky voice called for the dog from the hay barn. Behind the bales he could just make out the figure. He lifted his rifle, aimed – and took a shot at the silhouette hitting the figure square on the side of the head. Ha! He thought that will teach him a lesson…

I woke to the smell of breakfast cooking, but I would not be having any. I was unsure whether I had been seen or not. The inhabitants were awake and I could hear their chatter coming from the farm house. They would certainly have noticed the dog wandering round the yard while I was sleeping. I gathered myself together and called the dog. Someone was moving about out of sight in the yard. It wasn't a good idea to be caught resting here and I called again, 'Faith!' there was the sound of an iron gate closing and what sounded like the hiss of an air rifle. The dog came running from around the corner of the cow barn and I put her on the leash. She was limping; the bastard must have shot her. There was another hiss and I had an ache in one side of my head and I began to feel sick. As the trickle of sweat and drizzle ran down the side of my face I gathered my thoughts I took an unwary piss in the field that joined the barn. It was time to be moving.

I was sure to be invisible on my approach in the shadows but had to make sure I wasn't seen on my exit. I made my way down the dirt track quickly as I could, avoiding the inhabitants. I could hear the sound of dogs behind me snapping and gnarling having been let into the yard. I raced to the end of the track just in time to hear the roar of a tractor burst into life and start down the track. But by then I was on the road. I didn't want to stick around. I made my way hastily up the lane just as the tractor passed me, with the farmer shouting for me to 'get the fuck out of here!' and finally turning at the village green leading to the old turnpike, and staring me out.

I was on the road and free to do as I please. I forgot about our injuries and I took the road through some of the most affluent countryside on the Wirral. Here there were half million pound houses and golf courses, country cottages and on hundred acre farms. Here I had no friends as anywhere. An hour and five miles later I came upon a railway bridge and took shelter from the rain that was falling in a fine mist. It was the worst kind of rain soaking me through. The wind froze me as it ripped across the fields. I tried to make a cigarette but couldn't get my hands to work. I continued my journey on through the suburbia.

I was thinking about making my way to Parkgate at this point to pass by my girlfriend's house. The relationship I had with my girlfriend was like this; I had written to her all through my teenage years promising marriage and commitment but had bottled my chance at meeting up with her at sixteen. Three years later I had not forgotten her and still wrote to her when I needed a friend. Often I would think she would sometimes visit and sit in her car outside my home pretending to be waiting for someone. I had always thought it was me. Today did not seem like a good a time to show my face however. I had obsessed about my love for her in writing but I knew by our parting it was an unhealthy infatuation. I feared the town she lived in as much as her. As I came upon a turn in the road and Heswall, I was cursed with an inner turmoil. I could not find the purpose to confront her with the commitment I had made of us together. My doubts had got the better of me and I took a different turn. Fearing I could not face the good thing I had left behind all that time ago I turned around and went back towards the open countryside. I didn't recognize the place, and struck out in the direction of Hoylake.

As I walked I first began to lose my mind proper. I must have found some speed in my pocket while I was searching for money and taken it all, as I was weak and disorientated, exhausted even. On my approach to five ways roundabout I was certain I had been hit by a car. My dog was most certainly was, though she was unharmed. I had forgotten she was at my side when I crossed. As I walked I began to completely lose the reasonable intuitive of my mind. That is my thoughts where disordered and chaotic and I was rambling to myself incoherently aloud about all the things that didn't make sense. Moreover my failures. My temper boiled and I began making threats to the visions that confronted me. I swallowed my rage as best I could and carried on putting one foot in front of the other. Soon I had doubled back on myself and was heading towards Barnston again.

As I walked around in circles, the voices continued

to insult my sound beliefs. I answered the visions that appeared in my mind. 'Wanker! I chanted at myself, thinking of all the time I wasted before finally taking the chance to settle to speak to my girlfriend. I wondered if she would forgive me. It had been a long time gone. Intimacy was always the issue. I was always quite scared of the commitment I would have to make to someone one day. Its implications were strong in my mind. But to sacrifice my own being at the altar of the one I love was too great a gesture for me to carry out. Promises, I never could keep them. I tried to think back to when we first met. A flicker of the past passed through my mind; nine or ten maybe, chocolate brown hair, dyed and tied back in pigtails, strap sandals and knee length socks. The lane she lived on led up to a clearing in the woods. At night we would meet and swap an oral exam under the oak. I laughed; we had some fun back then. I must have been fifteen. Though six years of solitary sexual acts had not dampened my desire, my expression of it had been choked by my punishment. Six long years. I had hoped they would never end and that's the irony of it.

The rain was coming down in drenches as I and my dog trudged through the roads and on to Whitfield. I was avoiding coming into contact with others at this point. Taking to the footpaths and fields where I could to avoid civilization. I didn't want anyone to see me like this. The bedraggled appearance of the two of us stirred a mixture of emotions in those that came into our direction. One car of teenagers laughed and made jokes outside a restaurant.

Shane Leah

Others slowed their vehicles, staring at me. Some sounded their horn and waved. I had no idea why these people took an interest in me. I had hoped someone would stop and offer me some shelter from the elements by giving me a lift. None did. At one point I thought my father passed by but he didn't stop either. Naturally I thought I was being watched and began to look around myself. This made me look suspicious if I wasn't already a dead ringer for an omen of death and I became more hurried to get to my destination. The traffic got busier as I approached Arrow Park and the cemetery. I had family nearby and I was looking forward to seeing them so I could rest my weary legs. Us two recreants hooked a left and went towards Pensby. My aunt and uncle lived on a cul-de-sac here. As I walked up to their drive I thought I could hear the moans of burning passion coming from a window nearby. I rang the doorbell. There was no answer. I knocked and waited.

Mrs. Leigh was out getting the weekly groceries. At home her niece was checking out her housemother's porn. She had the morning to herself and was indulging. She did not expect any visitors. Suddenly a knock at the door startled her. Outside a rough cut figure loomed on the doorstep smoking. She did not want to answer. Pulling her gown on she trotted to the door, 'Wait a minute' she cried. She put on her slippers and looked through the frosted glass at the stranger outside. 'Who is it?' 'Shame,' came the reply. She had no idea who it could be, it certainly wasn't the postman. She gasped at the ghastly situation she found herself in.

DEAD CITY STREETS

'Oh, not today! She shouted from the other side of the door, and returned to hide her DVD's. When she looked out the window the figure was already leaving, tossing away a cigarette as he walked. She chased down the path to pick up the discarded butt shouting, 'We don't do that round here!' behind him as he walked away. As she closed the door she couldn't help but feel she knew him from somewhere.

Having not got an answer I turned in the direction I had come from and I walked past the Landican cemetery into Woodchurch and along Woodchurch road. Crossing at the flyover after a stop to pee I took a turn onto the pathway that leads you along the side of the motorway to Noctorum. I stopped opposite the Old Birkonians Football Club and looked across the far side of the motorway from my vantage point aloft the top of the rail bridge. From here I felt like I had come far enough. I could feel something waiting for me. I made a cigarette and let my dog off her leash to do her business in the bushes. A group of young lads came over the footbridge. They were first to introduce themselves and start conversation asking the dogs name. I told them it was Faith and they took a cigarette between them. They talked to me about a girl they knew, saying she was a slag and a whore and such like. I suspected a stolen love affair but they were adamant that they had not slept with her they told me she was much older and lived in Bidston. I laughed telling them they all were by the time you reached twenty one and they would be glad for any dirty old slag to swallow their grievance. They seemed worried at my response and talked amongst themselves for a minute before telling me I would get AIDS if I fucked her and then said goodbye. I finished my cigarette and watched them walk up the path away.

The rain had stopped falling and the temperature rose. My sodden clothes dried quickly in the sun as I walked up the hill towards Tam O'Shanter community farm, a petting zoo to all intents. On my entrance to the park I came across two women walking their dogs. That is one looked like a woman the other more like a man in drag. I ignored their presence and found a perch on an embankment, high above the park; here I decided to get some sleep if I could and took the dog's collar to let her roam around. When I woke, I was to have a discreet liaison with someone I had met that morning.

Laura was enjoying Christmas morning walking her two Great Danes in the park adjoining the Ladies golf course. She had come all the way from the village on the plain to see her cross-dressing uncle, who lived nearby and enjoy the spread put on by the club. While walking in the park, she and her uncle had caught sight of a homeless man and took pity on him. She chose to keep an eye out for him while he slept high above the green of the park on an embankment, all the while talking to her friends by mobile phone. Her uncle had nipped off to gather some provisions for the poor young man and his dog, a blanket, thermos and such like. While he slept she fussed his pet and fed it biscuits and let it run with her dogs in the wood. She could not be sure how long the man had been living like this. His dog seemed well fed and looked after as her uncle had pointed out, though she seemed quite exhausted. She wondered how far they had travelled and what for. Curious of his beginnings, she drew close to where he was resting and identified the dog as Faith, from her collar by his side, and they were from a nearby town. Though far away should they have walked here? As he began to stir, she retired to behind the bushes out of sight to phone the number on the collar, satisfied she could solve this young mans distress at this Christmas.

Several hours after reaching the park I was laying on top of the embankment with my eyes closed listening to a soft voice talk to another person or a dog. I was sure I could hear her talking about me and then to me. Her words were that of concern for someone less fortunate than herself. I could feel myself stirring and so sat upright. This was not the time or the place to get an urge. I rose to my feet to find another place to sit away from here. I made my way down the incline to the square and the park.

Here I listened intently trying to catch the words of her conversation from behind the bush to the side of me. I took a peep round the corner to see what she looked like. She was a good looking girl of about twenty two, blonde hair and blue eyes, tall and well turned out. Beautiful, even. Her two dogs were well groomed and you could tell looked after. She must be rich I thought, though it did not strike me to wonder if she was the whore I had been warned about by the boys in Noctorum. They had told me the prostitutes from the car wash lived in the vicinity. I couldn't think who she reminded me of, a movie star perhaps.

As I stared I noticed there was no one with her. At first it appeared she was talking to herself, or the birds before I saw she had a mobile phone in her hands. She was obviously a happy person, and as the dogs where fetching the stick she had thrown she looked right at me and smiled. I darted back in laughing to myself having been caught peeping. In my madness, desire stirred inside me. I tried to ignore it but my heart was racing. Knowing what I was about to do was dangerous I reached into my jeans and stroked my manhood. I was close to orgasm and pulled down my zipper, flopping it out thinking I needed to take a piss. A giggle came from behind the bushes, 'yeah, he's doing it' I thought she said into her mobile phone. I sensed the excitement of the situation, being exposed outside was erotic. I looked at the ugly old man then I considered the consequences of my intent. Putting it back away I took another peek of the girl. I would have loved to but something held me back... I thought, 'I must get out of here...'

I stood on my feet and was about to make my escape on a tangent when a man I had seen with her earlier came into view from the other side of the lawn. He was in a hurry and I realised the danger I was in. Not wanting to get arrested or embarrass myself further and I chose this as my time to leave. I started out from behind the bushes in a march, the dog following, so as to seem that I had only just chanced upon the place and walked away from him, towards her, at a pace. She stood, turned to me and said 'hello' as I passed. Surprised at her supposed recognition of me, I stopped a few paces past her and turned to see her smiling right at me. I paused for a moment waiting to see what direction the fat man in a dress would take then I made my approach cautiously not taking my stare from her eyes. Maybe she knows me I thought, but as I drew nearer she laughed and stared at the ground, then 'NO...I heard her say in a soft tone. As I drew close enough to touch she moved away and I felt two large strong hands take me by the shoulders and manoeuvre me away from her onto the lawn. The dog leash slipped out of my hands and I felt powerless over my direction. Behind me the fat man delivered me from fucking the whore. When I turned to face him he simply said 'No' and walked back to the girl. Shaken by the fear of having been caught committing a sexual offence I hurried off in the direction of the train tracks to hide.

I wanted to protest that I needed more than this. For good reasons nonetheless I left, I could see the headlines splashed across the tabloids. 'Homeless Schizophrenic Rapes Woman'. But I maintain she wanted it. I stopped again not far from the exit of the park to consider my feelings. I wanted to go back and ask the girl if she could give me a bed for the night. In my deranged condition I half believed she would, and did return after about thirty minutes with the excuse of finding my dog, only as I expected she was gone. I called for Faith, but she did not come and so I returned to the bottom of the hill to sob to myself. I, let alone my family would never forgive me for losing the only thing I had ever loved. As I sat moping over my loss a man called over to me asking if I had lost a dog. 'Yes, I replied. 'She's by the road, mate.' He said ('...fucking knobhead'). I raced down the hill avoiding the glare of the stranger and snatched the lead up off the floor. Further up the hill the odd couple were looking down talking animatedly as a great green tractor piled up the hill into town.

Having no reason to hang around I set off back down the hill in a panic and along the pathway to Woodchurch road. The traffic was heavy and I passed down all the roads I was familiar with, towards the city park. I had a friend there and planned to give him a call. First though I would need to eat and I went looking for a chip shop. Had I known that it was not just any Monday (which I didn't) but a bank holiday weekend at Christmas I would not have bothered trying to find a chip shop that was open because I couldn't. But did find a corner shop open by the park and so resorted to eating half a Jamaican ginger cake split between me and the dog.

Having finished our only meal in two days I sat on the benches watching faith explore the park while I chain smoked, eventually laying down and sleeping a while. I dreamt a wooden carousel was on the park lawn and soon young families were to be paying visits. It looked like a well crafted wooden flying saucer or a carousel closed for the winter. I walked around it to see what on earth it was and stepped inside. There was a bar and I ordered a beer and attempted to fit in to the scene. I was to have no such luck, I made idle conversation with the only other person in there besides the barman before being forced to leave by the incessant taunts of paedophilia I could hear from the only other punter there. I was sure it was him, though I knew my mind was unhinged. Before long the bloke behind the bar began joining in the taunts too. I felt like an Alien, I wasn't welcome anywhere in my condition and so I left the craft and wandered around the park looking for a place to lose myself before settling on the cricket pavilion to build a smoke.

My mind was feeling much better for the benefit of a dinner and I enjoyed the sunshine while lying on the cricket pavilion. Again I gradually dozed off and dreamed of my meeting with the girl at Bidston. I woke about two hours later because the temperature had fallen as the clouds formed overhead. Taking in my surroundings it appeared I had aroused some attention. Maybe it was anti vagrancy day in the park I didn't know but people all around where shouting obscenities in my direction. 'Nonce, beast, faggot! I could hear coming from all directions along with 'Go home John,' from behind. I didn't know whoever John was, and sat watching the dog chase other dogs while trying to get my head around my predicament and the abuse I perceived I was suffering, if I was this John. I didn't know. I thought no-one knew my name here but knowing I had no control over my nocturnal habits, especially under duress I chose not to stick around and moved through the gates to the far end of the park. I called on my friend.

In Newton, Gary had just woken and was planning his activities for the day. They usually involved cocaine and taking trips around town collecting money and dishing out the deals. Today would be no different, only he intended to enjoy it as much as anyone else. Looking out his flat window onto the park he could see the festivities had already begun as the carousel was here as every year, looking like a Stone Age spaceship. Later in the day he would be able to watch the children of the city immersed in play around the area, while imbibed adults drank themselves into a stupor and then sobered with a little help from him. Today would no doubt be the busiest of the year with all his friends and acquaintances making their way to his hallowed door in search of something to make the day swing. He was doing a line, the first of the morning when the buzzer rang out. Without looking to see who it was he pressed on the intercom and let the first customer of the day in.

My friend was a dealer. I buzzed his flat and waited. The buzzer went and I opened the door leaving the dog in the yard by the bins. Taking the 12 steps in four strides I reached the landing and entered. This place was dire. My own flat had a share of paraphernalia about the place but here it was stacked and cut and sorted. It was always a tense experience scoring. You never really knew the people, what they where capable of or how far they would go. I sat on a drum stool and asked him for an eighth of base which was cut and sorted in seconds then asked him something that had been on my mind for ages, I asked, 'Are you Gary Glitter?' In my psychoses I had thought he was, he certainly looked like him. There was no hesitation in his slowed reaction, I believe I scared him. This was a dodgy business and he was edgy enough without any pranksters knocking on his door, but it amused his humor and I think he soon saw the funny side. After all he was my hero. He recovered quickly as did I, by passing him a note, doing a line, begging a couple of joints worth and making my exit. Outside I laughed at my jibe. I had thought he was.

Outside it had gotten dark and the rain was falling again. I almost forgot the dog and walked into the road without her only to have to turn around. At first I was worried because she wasn't there. Fearing the worst I began to panic, skyrocketing my high into an acid trip. I brushed round the bushes to flush her out to no avail. I checked the car park to the front and then the back yard again, when she came from the direction of the road. With her being black could not see her at first in the dark and I walked out into the road, with her following me. Again she was nearly ran down and under the glow of the sodium lamp I grabbed hold of her leash and lead her off back to the park. I knew I should have chosen to go home now. I had, had my time and another night was going to be uncomfortable. I was on a super massive dose of uncut speed in freezing temperatures. It did occur to me to take the bus home from outside the flat, only I was reluctant to return to my home to what I knew and loved because it or I had to change.

I walked to the pond in the park and stepped over the fence. On the bandstand I cut a line and snorted it off the wall using a bus ticket I found on the path. My adrenaline coursed through my veins bringing a rush of energy that fixed me to the spot. I felt like I was going to faint. I stood rooted to the spot breathing deeply until I regained my composure. I had hoped for this to give me the energy to go on. But once the initial rush was over I crashed on the floor and my ideas went acid. There was no going home now.

I believe I then went on to spend an hour walking around and around the pond in the park rambling an incantation to myself in an effort to succeed in finding happiness. Love that is. I didn't mean to be ironic but I thought someone would be looking out for me at least. I could not see reason to be satisfied is what the problem appeared to be. There could be something more certain and real around the next corner was my philosophy. Having finished my ritual I lit a joint, lifted my dog over the fence and made my way into the dark towards one of the many entrances.

My mobile had run out of charge and I couldn't get the time. Thinking it was late I tried to find some shelter. At one of the entrances I found a derelict scout hut and clambered through the bushes to get to it. It was a burnt out shell and only the porch had survived the fire, this is where I was to build a joint. The rain was drenching me in this little cubby-hole. I struggled to put the Rizlas together without them blowing away or getting wet. I certainly could not manage to burn weed into the half rolled papers and gave up in frustration. I had my pipe handy however and set about getting my fix that way. Not satisfied I added some of the powder had just picked up and set about smoking that too.

Now, whereas in the afternoon I had been feeling struggling both physically and mentally, my episode in the park was to tip the scales. I hadn't tried smoking this gear before and as my mind was unhinged anyway I was in for a rough ride through my soul once more. The intoxicating smoke slept into my lungs and I stared out across the railings and into the dark of the park. My eyes glazed over and I began to hallucinate. The cold and rain could not stop me slipping off into my own world once more. I thought of home and all it meant to me. I thought of past loves and labors, friends and enemies. What did it all mean I thought to be out here in the thick of it when I have somewhere to go? I was so intent on my pipe dream that I didn't notice the police turn up right in front of me. I managed to make a cigarette while they sat in their car. Probably looking for a suspicious character hiding in some bushes I thought to myself, chuckling. I didn't think they could see me from where they were and so I kept my head down.

I watched commuters race through the rain and showers, hurrying to their homes. I wondered when

I would be returning to mine. Some stopped and talked to the policeman. They were certainly looking for me. The woman pointed to the pond where I had just come from and I hoped to become invisible. I hid in the dark of the alcove not stirring and waited for them to leave. Once they had I made some preparations to stay the night as it was too cold and wet to consider the journey this late in the evening. I would need to stay warm and dry.

I climbed into the burnt out shell that once was the scout hut through a broken window and had a rummage about looking for something to cover myself with. On the floor there was some wet carpet amid all the fallen debris. Not that I thought. Then looking above me I discovered a discarded duvet and pillow in the rafters above the entrance. Taking them down I found them to be dry. My mood lifted immediately and I clambered back outside to the porch to bed down for the night.

The bed linen had lice all over it but I still wrapped it around me to cut out the chill of the wind and built another pipe. I sat leaning against the wall taking hits and trying to find the comfort zone I had before the police had arrived. As I sat my mind began to wander again. This time I considered all the bad things that I had in my life. My fear of being alone, the worry for the future, the injustices I had faced and the subject of my sexuality. All of this enraged me and I nearly bit off my tongue, shouting at the accusations of my hallucinations. I was also cold and this made my temper flare too. I could not get comfortable. Maybe in the summer camping under the stars would be a good idea but tonight a few hours was a matter of life or death. I considered my options and chose to set alight the bed linen hoping the burning flames would give me some warmth. This was a stupid idea as I needed warmth and shelter from the rain. The burning embers of the blanket only smoldered and didn't catch light, sending out noxious fumes all around my camp choking me and attracting the attention of passers-by. I had no choice but to leave this place and find another doss. The dog was somewhere nearby but I had not seen her in half hour or more. I occasionally caught what I thought to be a glimpse of her running by me in the dark but I was uncertain and confused as the toxic effect of the drugs took hold and bent my mind and vision.

Inside his flat Gary watched a TV game show. He wondered what condition his friend was in outside in the park. He seemed to be in a bad way, eyes wild and agitated. Scared of something perhaps. The carousel was still on the lawn of the entrance to the park, thought the visitors had all gone home. While his back was turned a news flash came on the screen alerting the viewers to the elderly and alone at Christmas. He wondered where his insane friend would be keeping this Christmas. He picked up the phone and made the call.

I still had not taken the leave to go home but instead was looking for another doss. I chanced upon a series of disused anti aircraft gun brackets and took a chance to whether the storm here inside the towers that once held them. First I lifted Faith into the tower above my head then pulled myself into the den. I was not the only recent visitor to this place. There was evidence of pot smokers and a recent fire. I bedded down here as best I could. I smoked and dreamed the worst of the thunder and lightening through to the end. Faith whimpered and complained at having been away from home so long. I smoked and dreamt of all that was not. I considered my ambition to be here with nothing, why I had come and what for. It seemed I was searching for someone unique. A special bond like that of a mother. Maybe that was whom I missed so much. I did not want to be alone at this time of year but nonetheless I had made it this way. This epiphany was a revelation to me and I gathered myself together frantically and jumped down the hole in the floor, hitting my head on the balustrade as I fell. It knocked all sense out of me. I staggered about the floor weeping and delirious clutching my head in my hands. I had to kneel on the floor for a few minutes to shake off the ache in the side of my head. I lifted the dog down from the tower with great difficulty, dropping her in the process and then, holding my head I walked towards the orange streetlights.

I got lost in the dark and it took ages for me to find my way out of the park. Under an orange streetlamp by the gates I asked a passing stranger for the time. It was early evening about eight o'clock, a lot earlier than I expected. There was time to make it home even if I walked and thus I could take my time. I stopped at Gary's again. I buzzed and entered as normal, joining him in the flat. He wasn't amused to see me return. I greeted

DEAD CITY STREETS

him and asked if he could see his way to lending me some change so I could get home. Again his mood was one of caution. But he opened a jar of coppers and removed the lid. He asked the fare and I guessed a figure, you sure any trains run today? He asked, 'Yeah,' was my reply, not sure what I was doing here for the second time in one day. Throwing the coins at me he was about to see me swiftly out the door when I delivered the punch line, 'can I have some weed as well, for these...' I handed him a scrapbook of verses I had made myself and carried with me for inspiration, bound with duct tape. He didn't look at it and instead set about calling one of my friends to tell him I was making a nuisance of myself. I didn't wait for him to finish the call. I made my joint and went, leaving the poems behind.

I walked into the city centre towards the Christmas lights. The traffic was as busy as any other time of the year even though everything was shut. I answered the voice of my conscious telling me I was rich. I reveled in the thought of being a cash millionaire, 'I'm Slim Shady!' I shouted out loud to myself puffing on my joint, laughing. A passing stranger looked at me stunned and afraid, - I thought I was. I made my way into the city centre and stopped for a drink. I asked if I could bring the dog inside and the bartender obliged. I sat drinking my beer quietly, listening to two young men joke about their day. I had no money but I ordered another drink and when asked for payment I bluffed it by asking if the bartender knew who I was, 'just this one time then.., he said. I was certain I was a famous writer. I wasn't sure, but I could have been. I was keen to tell the bartender how important I was in the industry but he was too 'up' on the social makeup of occasional drinkers in this town and avoided my efforts to engage him in conversation. By now the dog was getting restless and looking for a place to shit, her whimpering told me it was time to go.

Immediately on stepping outside, the dog took a turd in the doorway. I dragged her away from the scene as dog owners do when they're pet takes a dump in town, the dog whining and grunting as the choker got tighter on her neck. Hastily we power walked through the city centre to Central station to make my journey home to recuperate but that was unlikely on Christmas Eve. Upon reaching the station and finding it shut, I took a route back into town looking for a phone box with which to call my dad and ask him to pick me up. I couldn't find one that wasn't vandalized and ended up walking back round town in circles for what seemed to be hours, taking in all the places I was familiar with. I decided to pass by my uncle Kenneth's house.

Ken was waiting for his wife to finish getting ready for their Christmas dinner at a local restaurant. His daughters were already putting on their coats and combing their hair. In the dark of the street a shadowy figure passed in front of the house, stopping to peep through the curtains. He continued to watch 'Who Wants to be a Millionaire' and snacked on chocolate Brazils in front of a blazing fire. A knock came at the door. He could

DEAD CITY STREETS

see who it was and shouted to his wife to answer it and continued to watch the TV. A few moments passed until one of his daughters raced to look through the eyelet in the door and shouted back that it was some strange man. 'Don't let him in! He shouted and popped another chocolate Brazil into his jaw's laughing. 'He deserves her!'

I waited for an answer outside Kenneth's for a few minutes but I could hear the conversation inside and chose to continue walking and save the humiliation of asking for help. I just wanted to get warm as the temperature was falling rapidly. I kept moving, I walked through Wallasey and on to the ferry. I walked my dog to the bus terminal by the ferry and sat down. The dog had gotten tired and whimpered in protest at being kept away from home so long. She was limping having walked so far and had not been fed and watered. We were both exhausted. I reassured her with a fuss and made a cigarette with what little tobacco I had left, offering the dog the rest thinking she may eat it. We had to keep moving if we were to stay alive. We walked up the promenade as far as the pier as the wind blew a gale. I had been here before hoping to meet with some person or thing that would give me a reason to live. Again I was to meet with disapointment. There was nothing here for me. I considered the purpose of my journey. Gazing out across the river I tried to lose myself in emotion. I had nothing with which to share my experience of life. I had tried all the places where I believed I had someone only to be turned away in detest. I really was on my own. I stood and continued my walk.

I kept to the shadows on my walk through the industrial estate. The dog in front of me all the way, we crossed the road into the housing estates and avenues of the city centre. In front of me a young woman was hagging her trade along the ball park to the side of the old towerblock. I crossed the road to avoid her, not wanting to show my face. As I passed on the other side, she crossed the road and followed me onto the council offices. I thought she called my name and I looked behind me. I recognized her from the ladies golf club, or at least I thought she was. She wore her hair up, with flashes of pink and blonde platted round the side of her head and a pink tracksuit. I continued to walk, ignoring her presence and when I looked behind again she had disappeared. I wondered what I had done. Could she be a whore? Almost certainly, I realized I may be in some danger when the stranger that had passed me by the park wielded a Stanley blade at me and so I picked up the pace out of the city and back to the park. All the time the warning of the boys in Noctorum attempted to enter my conscious thought. I dismissed it as paranoid and entered central park from the north east gate to lose the attention. I stumbled through the park in a nervous hurry until I reached the other side and then fled as quickly as possible as far as Egremont and onto the unassuming bar facing the sea front.

I bought another small pouch of tobacco and two bottles of wine a few yards down the road from where I had stopped and sat on the beach in front of the Brass Balance staring out into the black of sea. I was too shy to go into the pub and ask for the use of a corkscrew to open the bottle of wine and so smashed the neck off the bottle by striking it against the sea wall and drinking the contents and glass shards in all. It tasted just like wine always had, dry and sour. Voices called from the 'Balance and I kept to the shadow cast by the lights against the small sea wall. A taxi arrived and amidst some shouting and exclamation of insults a man left in his ride, taking a Moses basket with him. The lights outside the bar soon switched off and I made off down the promenade and back towards Egremont, stopping at Vale Park to settle into my emotions again. The lights in the bedroom of a house above and behind me, mistook my eyes for her beloved while I smoked several cigarettes in the dark. The air was fresh and silent as the tide swelled into the channel; I put a foot forward in the direction of home for the umpteenth time that night.

We walked down four bridges road taking in the derelict dock buildings and swing bridges. I had always wanted to know the history of this place, the purpose of the quayside and the reason for the sunken vessels. There were not any streetlights here so the headlights of passing cars blinded me on their approach. The rain drenched down on top of me soaking me in its deluge as I crossed the dock. To my right was a fifteen meter steel box section that appeared to be part of a prefabricated something or other and blocked the access to the East Float. Ahead of me was an old swing bridge, once the entrance to Wallasey Dock. Curious of its purpose and keen to escape the deluge of rain, I climbed the stairs and broke the lock by twisting the latch off with a discarded screwdriver by the wayside of the door. Once inside I let the dog wander round the levers and apparatus whilst I scrubbed at the windows to get a better look at the float below me. Through the grime of the city on the windows, the dark of the clouds overhead and the drenching rain pouring down now as hail upon the East Float, I could not see further than the road below. I walked around the room and found a large hole in the floor through which I could see the passing cars and Lorries. Faith joined me and almost fell through it in her haste to explore the new den. I tied her lead to one of the levers and scraped enough tobacco together to roll a cigarette.

Sitting down, I felt the peace of a tranquil melancholy come over me as I listened to the hail falling on the felt roof and the smell of the passing traffic. Faith wagged her tail and shook herself in an exclamation of joy as I spoke to her to tell her we were going home soon. She obviously could not wait and whined at my taunt of seeing mother. Below people passed and cars honked they're horns as they clattered over the bridge. All around me were levers and cylinders of pneumatic fluid, barrels of oil and a thick layer of dust. I picked up a log file and read the entries. It seemed the last time the bridge was raised was the previous year on New Years Eve to let a tug boat enter the dock.

Looking around at the many levers and buttons something took hold of me. I don't know whether it was a devious cruelty or just an experimental idea but I chose to pull a few and see what happened.

DEAD CITY STREETS

At first nothing moved, though the traffic did stop flowing and so I pressed another green button and soon the traffic was building up right outside. For a few brief moments I panicked thinking I would be found up in this loft tower and be in trouble and so pressed all the buttons again hoping it would allow the traffic to flow again. Sure enough the traffic began to inch forwards again and the congestion eased. Amused at my discovery I pressed the buttons again and pulled on one of the levers just as soon as the congestion had cleared. I looked outside to see if anything was moving but all's I could see was pitch darkness and the red light of the traffic signal.

I moved across the floor to the other side and peered out across the bridge to see if it was moving but I couldn't see a thing and so went back to the levers and pulled on all of them. I felt what I thought was wind shaking the loft housing and the squeal of brakes. Frightened, I poked my head around the door to see the bridge had risen to a ninety degree angle and some cars had stopped on the Woodside bank. Fortunately the traffic signals all around were on red and so my fear dissipated and I returned inside to replace everything as I found it. Having done so and the traffic had started moving again we left the hut behind and clattered down the stairs and away. As I crossed the bridge and onto Woodside with Faith on her lead a car parked at the side of the road appeared to have been in a collision but there was no-one around to witness it other than an angler pitched on Wallasey Dock who watched me pass with a few choice words.

I was in town now at Woodside. The bar there had been left unoccupied a long while now and I found an open door to the back of a bar and entered into a needle strewn room. The discarded sharps cracked underfoot and I beat a hasty retreat back to the entrance. I sat on the stairs and considered my next steps. It was too cold to stay out here I knew I had to return home.

As I was sat in the doorway at the side of the Woodside, a car stopped nearby and the occupants waved in my direction, calling me over. I went to them to ask for help. I thought it was my uncle and aunt come to help me out but they ignored my tap on the window. I waited for a response but they drove off smiling. It was a real strike to the gut to be treated this way. I had given up on finding any help here and when I looked down into the murky waters of the Mersey, wondering if I would suffer less if I was to throw myself off the ferry wall. My depression did not go unnoticed by a passer by who shouted 'Oi, in my direction, Do it!' I laughed, in the face of suicide I had been amused by this stranger. I tried to hide my mood, but my situation was untenable I wanted to go. I leant over the barrier to see if I could make it happen for myself once he had gone, but couldn't. The dog would have followed me and I thought and my family would not miss me but Faith. I clambered back over. I could not do it, even if it was to save my dog from the same fate as me. Strangely the contemplation of death did make me happier.

For a few moments, I watched the step of the tide

swell below the sea wall under the ferry dock. It seemed to want me to be drawn to it, maybe the river wanted my life I thought. I contemplated the Grace's on the far bank, then turned back to face the bus stop. I wondered where I might go next.

Taking to the street again I came to rest at the opposite side of the Woodside pub. Here I sat in the doorway waiting for the chance to get home. I was hungry and tired and searched in my bag for some sustenance. All I had to eat though was half a bag of sugar and some leftover ginger cake crumbs. I sat in freezing temperatures in the doorway looking blankly across at the opposite wall thinking something would be along any minute to help me out. It didn't come. In the grip of starvation I made my way to the taxi rank just a few yards along the road and ordered a cab. The office was warm and I felt grateful for the kindness of the operators for heating the place, I told them so and smoked the dregs of my collected cigarette dimps. When it arrived and I started my journey home the distance I had covered in the past two days stripped back as I traveled. The streets I had roamed through were dead and listless. Nothing stirred in the empty soul of the Wirrals' housing estates. When I arrived home I signed the cheque Sonny Bono and retired to the house to sleep.

Amelia, my youngest sister, was asleep in bed when the front door slammed shut, waking her from a nightmare. The previous day the phone had rang all afternoon with people searching for the whereabouts of her brother. He was in some sort of trouble, but her parents would not inform her as of to what. She had her own suspicions; he had either gotten arrested or died somewhere. All the chaotic excitement happening around her had given her a bad dream about his whereabouts. She was sure she had seen him on the television in her dream as a game show host, on a program called 'Bet Your Life,' where he interviewed his family and friends about his own life history. His replies however were comic book. She was sure she could hear him now giving a loaf of bread a good talking to downstairs. 'Fuck you, you little slut! I'm gonna fuckin' kill yer! Sssssllutttt ! Then cursing himself under his breath to control his temper. She crept out of bed and downstairs to see if it was him. From the landing she could see him buttering up an iced bun with the intent of killing it, or so it seemed. He was threatening to kill the slag as he called it. Screaming at it in a serious hushed tone that it had not had his children and wasn't welcome at his home. More amused than anything she returned to bed, leaving her mother a note that Shane was home.

Back home I crashed on the sofa. I was exhausted and dozed off without thinking of feeding the dog. In the morning my sister walked in and immediately started shouting the odds on where I had been and the whereabouts of the dog. Telling me my mother had been looking for me she hurriedly woke her to let her know the news. I had no time for her concern though. I simply rolled over and went back to sleep. My mother arrived downstairs a few minutes later and erupted in anger to find me asleep on the couch. I blazed back and retired upstairs to my box room to sleep. My mother followed screaming that my father wanted to see me too and that I was to find professional help for my alleged problems, in the New Year. I didn't understand what she meant. Why did I need help? I thought that I was just having a rough few weeks.

I slept and dreamed of how I used to be. I dreamt I was in my old room. The fun I had in my old room making plans and creating music. I loved my old space in the world, I had it just as I wanted it only then I had moved out to the flat to make a new start. It was more like a false start. I got to my feet and looked out the window. The street was active as ever. Outside my father pulled up in his car and came to the front door. I was glad to see him as I wanted to tell him about my adventure. I heard him come up the stairs and go into my brothers' room. I expected him to come into mine. I waited listening to his voice emanating from the next room expecting him any minute to burst into my room and have a go at me. But he didn't.

I left my room and went into my brothers to speak to him. I paused a hello, to which he replied but then as I went on to talk to him he ignored me and only replied to the comments of my brother's game play. He was in a bad mood you could tell. I clamored for his attention asking questions and telling him my story. At one point I thought he answered me but he was talking to my brother. Then with a start he said goodbye to my brother and left the room... Me and my father had not seen eye to eye for a long time because of my drug habits. He had not forgiven me today. Years of drugs and gratuitous addiction to pornography had driven a clear distance between us. He had no time for me any more.

Dad was downstairs now and I could hear him talking to my mother telling her that he wanted me home tomorrow then he left slamming the door behind him. I went downstairs myself to speak to my mother. I asked her why they where all having a go at me. She ignored me too and continued to race about the place doing the housework. I protested at her attitude and raised my voice. She erupted in a vehement slaughter cutting me down to earth. She told me in one statement. 'You need to see a doctor.' Did I? The gravity of my encounter in the park grew on me and I wondered what she meant. I recoiled at the accusation and returned to my room. What had I done to deserve this I thought? I sat on the bed staring at the skirting board. I was in a panic and I shook with fear. Something was wrong even I had to admit I was acting strangely. This vision of myself cleared my head for a few minutes before my conscience took over again with its endless dialogue.

I woke to the lime green color of the room. I hated this box room, the color of the walls was awful and it was crammed with prams and pushchairs, old cupboards and boxes of disused junk. It was no wonder I could not sleep soundly here, I wanted my old room, the one I dreamed of, back off my sisters. But I would have to be leaving sooner than that. My head was clouded by dreary thoughts of what may have been had I just lived my life differently. I wrestled with the rational narrative of my mind as I lay in my pit. The hallucinations I was having made me cuss and flinch on my own beliefs. And I had some strange ones. I had gotten it into my head for some time that I was a world famous rock star that had been cheated of his wealth after a recording deal. I had told everyone about this and I certainly believed it. Most people kept clear of me for some time however and this is how I came to be estranged from my group of friends. I had not missed them, although I had attempted to get in touch. They were all to make an appearance today.

Martin had arrived outside his grandmothers home to speak to one of his family members, Paul. They discussed the day's events and the Christmas festivities and of course they're insane friend, Shane. He had been acting erratically for some weeks now and they had written him off as a lost cause. The cause of all this drama, as they well knew was his love affair with his young girlfriend. They did not wish him any harm but he had had it. When she finally told him to go, his mind split up into a thousand tiny fragments of dissident rage and humiliation. They had mocked his beliefs and ambitions and desires' to love and be loved,' as he could not compete in the band and was better off alone. They didn't think it, they knew it... As they spoke a Landrover pulled up outside his house. Out stepped a tall blonde woman who went to the back of the wagon and lifted out his dog Faith, wrapped in a blanket. They were ashamed at the possibility of his dog's death, as even though they knew the state he was in, losing his dog would shake him up, like last time. They both knew this was they're chance to tell him exactly what they thought of his attempts to take his girl as his own, as well as a control freak could. Shane's mother stepped outside at this point and called to them, asking if they would take him somewhere. Martin couldn't wait to stir up trouble, in an instant he was on the doorstep ready to take his piece of meat.

There came a knock at the door. My mother answered and I heard the voice of a so called friend Martin. Footsteps came up the stairs to the landing and in through my door. I was on the bed. He asked me where I had been and told me they had all been out looking for me. I doubted he had, I knew he would of just sat off somewhere. He invited me out, I declined the invitation saying I was too fucked up but he persisted and I gave in and left without changing. We went out to the car and he took me on a journey around the 'Port taking in all his friends on the way. The journey seemed an act of humiliation. Everyone said bad things about me calling me John, one of his friends spat at me.

He dropped me off at home about half an hour later. Here another friend, Paul, pulled me to one side and gave me a talking to about my complaints about the way I was being treated. I believed I had every right to complain, I was being walked on like a doormat, challenged in everything I had believed in and committed to. I refused to back down from my position and settled to speak again later. But we would not.

I returned to the house and sat in front of the television. The programs all seemed to be referring to me like there was a videophone connected between us. I answered their questions and replied to their requests; I thought I was a star. I changed channel to watch a music awards ceremony. Here I began to get into my hallucinations enjoying the moment I received my first Grammy award for greatest ruddy pop star in the world. I let out a cheer. My mother looked in and shook her head at the sight of me doing my acceptance speech and walked out. I had lost it. I however, could not see past it.

My mother made a phone call. Soon after my father arrived again and scorned at me asking how I was. I mumbled a reply and he left the room to speak to my mother. I was worried I was in some serious trouble. A few minutes passed and they returned. They told me a social worker would be to see me and would find me a hospital bed once into the New Year. I wondered what for, and protested for my freedom but agreed to go, to spare a furious argument. That settled the row and I was given some pills to take off the doctor. I swallowed them all and settled to lie in front of the TV all day. Only my mother refused to let me, saying she had visitors and I should go to my room. I went, to get away from the patronizing old bag. I ran a bath and relaxed in its heat, I was glad to be home though my family and friends could go screw themselves up the wall. Soon I would be admitted but until then

I could be sure I was not alone.

Anita called the boys from outside. 'What's been goin' on,' is what she wanted to know. None had a good answer. I was behaving strangely they had to admit that, but for why they had no idea. She asked the question she dreaded about his comments and beliefs, what did he mean? Paul had an answer, 'Drugs, is all he said, messed himself up.' 'Ah, ok then she said, but Anita wasn't satisfied with the answers she was getting and invited them to talk some more later. Something was afoot and she was a dangerous woman when the chips were down. She was going to find out the truth.

Just at that moment another friend Sim, screeched to a halt outside his friends. Immediately he demanded to know what was going on. He had a good mind to give him a fucking good thrashing for the trouble he had stirred up over the past few days and weeks. Now his friends were asking questions. What the fuck had he been doing? Some shit he bet.

Paul and Martin laughed at the scene that was playing out. It was a soap opera gone nuts. Any minute now the police would be along to arrest everyone.

Sure enough they were

Howie, one of his friends knew what was going on. He had received a call from a concerned friend and he arrived soon after to calm things down. It was him who suggested they call a doctor. He had seen this before.

I was told to go inside and wait for news. What news? I thought. Soon I was moved on to Sim's. I sat in his kitchen trying to make idle conversation with my host. He growled at me that I shouldn't be trying to make small talk with him. Slamming his fist on the work surface he turned his back on me and left me sitting alone while he spoke to his wife in the living room. Suddenly my breathing became heavier and I was choking on each breath, like I had swallowed my tonsils. Sam returned to the kitchen to find my huddled up in a heap over the kitchen worksurface. He raised his eyebrows called my name then opened the door and asked me to leave.

I thought I was dying, but no-one seemed to care.

Chapter 3

At Home

Later that day the doctor and psychologist arrived and listened to my concerns and threats of suicide. I told them of my loneliness and the competition I had to put up with as friends cheated me of lovers and friends. I told them of reaching rock bottom and losing the will to live because I had been cheated by the object of my affection. I told them of the incessant insults and perverted ideas that my mind kept forcing on me. Telling me all of the things I would never condone. I told them of my delusion, that I was a famous rapper and what the lyrics of my favorite artiste meant to me, though they were totally fallacious. They suggested that my sexuality was up for debate by my closest friends which offended me, but did not convince me. After everything I told them of, the doctor would ask how all this made me feel and I would reply that life was shit and not worth living.

We took a break and the doctor spoke to my parents. I could hear them talking in hushed tones in the kitchen about what to do with me. I sat despairing at my grief wanting to be comforted. I rolled a cigarette and waited. They returned from the kitchen and announced that there were no beds at the hospital and I could not be admitted until the New Year. Until then I was to take the prescribed medication and wait for my assessment. The initial diagnosis was I had suffered a complete and acute nervous breakdown. What was making me suffer? I didn't know.

My friends spoke to my mother. None could explain my questions or insults, my responses to they're conversations when out of earshot. Was I being crooked or had I done something wrong? None had a story. My youngest sister Amelia, sat rooted to the spot amongst all the heated discussion watching TV. 'Guess he has then, said Thomas. At last! Said the Fat Controller.

Chapter 4

Liverpool Gig

Liverpool was cold, dark and wet. I had come here in the evening on the bus to have a quiet drink and get away from myself and the pressure I was under. The streets were not busy as like every other New Year's Eve because it was bank holiday Monday. I moved through town quickly not waiting for traffic to stop before crossing roads. On reaching Lime Street I turned into the nearest bar to escape the rain that hailed down upon the city. I was glad to get that first fresh cold pint down me in the warmth of familiar surroundings. I settled by a window and gave thought to my motives for being here.

The reason I was still able to walk around freely was my hospital bed had been blocked, and my doctor and social worker could not admit me for assessment. I was overjoyed when the social worker told me; it was like escaping the hangman's noose. I got excited at the thought of evading the authorities like I was a Robin Hood figure, making a stand against the intellectual elite telling them I was greater in mind and spirit. I had taken the new medication after they had left though, hoping it would give me some clarity over my thoughts and their direction. It did and I became self assured that I was not at all unwell. In fact I had never felt better and I acrimoniously denied any faults in my reasoning and behavior. I was insulted by the suggestion that I was anything other than slightly perplexed and angry at the situation I found myself in at home and in love, blaming my mother and siblings and friends for my chaotic rages and the whispered taunts that came from me answering the voices that insulted me and wound me up.

So I had been and still was to an extent unwell. I had also become convinced that I was a world famous pop star and that everyone recognized me as such. The real problem though was I had mistakenly come to the conclusion I could not be loved. I believed I had failed in every relationship I had ever had. Be them members of the opposite sex or otherwise. I couldn't even make my mother happy. Every girlfriend I had ever had, cheated on me with my friends or fancied the pants off my brothers or where taken from me by some gorgeous gangster lothario with whom I could not compete or challenge. The result being I got used and abused. The subject of my sexuality and preference was up for discussion by friends and family and my confidence was drained.

My loss of confidence with women caused me endless bouts of sulking about not being able to communicate my needs to the opposite sex. My mother had worn down what little belief I had left in myself by forcing her criteria for a suitable candidate on me. I know it was only her concern that was showing but still it put me under pressure to find a soul mate, who was not to be forthcoming. It drove me spare and I acted like a teenager. I had become cynical and haunted by its heavy hand on my shoulder, making me look deep inside myself at my own isolation from the experiences of my friends, all of whom managed lasting relationships or sexual advances I would have paid for but couldn't afford.

This was my second time round so to speak, as there had been a period of celibacy between 17 and 20 where I never even spoke to a girl other than my mother and other close acquaintances. I had blown my chance at every interval stage by not being able to commit or failing to be satisfied emotionally, or to fail to satisfy. It was a hard luck story that only a student's life could bestow upon you, round the clock celibacy.

My new found perspective however, had determined me to change. The changes going on in my brain had given me a new chance to rediscover myself and I was looking for a new understanding. (Albeit a psychotic one with which I would continue to struggle). My meeting with the dog walkers in the park had stirred my desire and I was steering a new direction in my sex life. Here on a quiet Monday evening I could easily pick up something strayed from home looking for some casual first time encounter. I finished my pint and went in search of the next bar looking for the answers. I traveled through town looking for the Bar-Bar but could not find it and settled to stop at the back of a fire station and have a smoke.

I was unfamiliar with the layout of Liverpool (and still am though I go their often enough), and I had no idea of my whereabouts. I built a pipe from a can and honked on it till I choked. This weed was fucking good. It hit all the parts of you it should, sending a deep seated chill through me that felt like I was home and dry. I felt comfortable sitting here admiring the night sky and the tranquil hush of the city winding down from a year of decadence. To be here alone on the birth of the year 2000 was a burn and I had no qualms about my future prospects in the year ahead, however dire they may be. In fact I was looking forward to it.

After half hour of taking in the ambience of the city I gathered my parts together and set off back into town. I walked down Slater Street, looking for the prostitutes hanging outside the garage. I would of paid for sex (except for within a relationship), but just looked for one I may like the look of. Like the girl in the park. It was likely I would find her here. Some jeered across the road, mocking my look. More scared than embarrassed, I pressed on to the next bar, The Albert.

Sim was spending the night in Liverpool after being chucked out by his partner. He had taken his place at the bar in the Albert and was talking to the barmaid about his problems at home. Across the bar at the other end was his nemesis, Paul. His stare threatened to unnerve him as he spoke. They had a history he could not escape - a family tie that had not been respected. He avoided his attention by skulking behind the bar and the person sat next to him. A stranger approached the bar and ordered a drink; he was rough looking and dressed all in grey. He seemed high on something and the barmaid didn't think twice about short changing him. Turning back to Sim she offered him a drink. 'Thanks, he said, can you afford to? I can't she replied, he paid for It.' nodding towards the stranger. They laughed - Sim just hoped the character had not recognized him.

It has been said to me since that it was a gay bar, it was certainly a rough place but that didn't perturb me any I just wanted a drink. I settled amongst the regulars to sup my pint. Looking around I could see a few familiar faces from my past, or at least I thought so. Characters that I would have had been identified as being gay. With my new mind I recognized that I had an agenda within the gay arena, that being my sexuality was open to question. Especially in a place like this. It would have made my mother happy if I was to come out as being gay and for the duration of mine own opinion I was in the right place. I felt familiar with this place. Like I had been here before. I neglected to talk to my friends at the bar (I had seen them but not recognized them in this place) and sat drinking my pint and taking in the surroundings before making my way back to the street.

Where to go, what to do? I had no idea and it was still early. I fumbled about outside the Albert considering my options not knowing whether to go this way or that. I took a walk round the deserted streets of the New Year Eve looking for opportunity to strike. I had just a few more pounds in my pocket and was unsure of whether to take the train home or have another drink somewhere. I chose to have a drink and made my way back to Lime Street and the Duke. As I passed by what I thought to be the Adelphi Hotel I looked in and caught sight of a scantily clad woman, bikini, heels and hair. Tits, arse and legs. I stopped and helped myself to an eyeful and what I liked. Making my way up the steps to the entrance to get a better view, two bouncers closed in on me and asked for my membership. I told them I just caught sight of what they had in there and asked if I could go in. One asked me how much money I had and took a fifteen pound tip to let me in. Thrilled, I hastened into the bar area and ordered a drink.

Anne was working late at the strip bar. She had come from the Albert down the road, on a request from her manager who ran all the bars she worked in. She didn't want to work that night, really she wanted to be at home with her two cats watching TV. She had worked here before the authorities shut it down in the eighties, as a dancer. She had some regrets now about that. The hedonism of the eighties had taken its toll on her future and she was disappointed to be here again. Her melancholy was obvious to the stranger that walked in, whom she recognized from the Albert, as he immediately attempted to chat her up. He must have been having a laugh, what with her reputation and age before her in this place. She waited for him to ask where he could get shag, but it seemed he just wanted to talk. All life's big questions were extolled as he spoke. With even bigger answers, she was captivated by his enthusiasm for learning about life in adversity and her mood lifted as he queried her about her own life. It was like he cared. Fat chance she thought, but he was soon encouraging her to take up a new vocation. Maybe go to college, write a story, become a nurse. A nurse? He was having a laugh. But she had made up her mind. No longer would she give fate a chance. She gave the man a pint on the house and announced to the bar manager that she was going home.

The stripper had finished her performance and I was talking to the girl behind the bar and one or two other punters when the manager of the establishment approached me. He looked a lot like Sim. Asking my name he queried my thoughts about the bar and asked for my membership. I told him I was very happy to of found it and I was unable to pay for a membership today. He laughed at the rebel nature of the bouncers letting me in for a tip and told me I could stay till members only at eight o'clock unless of course I wanted to become a member. He was a friendly guy though and allowed me to stay.

The barmaid pulled me a pint and saw to it that the machine would accept my payment and give me cash back on my card. She asked me how long I had been in Liverpool. I told her I had only come across for the night and was looking for a new watering hole and discover my new self. She handed me my drink and invited me to come along again the following evening for the opening night on New Year's Day it was on her. I felt cared for here. Like all my real friends had spent there lives in a seedy nightclub I had never discovered until now. I chatted aimlessly to the barmaid. I felt a mood of hurt and rejection but here there seemed to be some security to be had. Like talking to a caring parent. She did, it seemed and I was glad to be having a good time for once.

I finished my drink and ordered another. A coke was all I could afford, though cocktails and cola came with lemon slices. Covered in what I assumed to be some narcotic substance. I tucked in to the flesh of the lemon and sipped my cola, amused at the cheek. The joint was winding down and I would soon have to be on my way. I wanted to stay and see the strippers but only had enough money for the train ride home. I swirled my drink round and looked deep into it wishing the staff would say I could stay longer. I ordered another coke with lemon, and settled to prepare to leave. My emotions took a dip knowing I would have to leave this great night behind. Within minutes I was asked to leave, I left my pop and walked out to the street.

Alan was having a late night drink before returning to his hotel. Outside the city was winding down from a hectic year of deviance. His reading material was a statistical analysis of breeding programmes and fish stocks. It was boring and he would of much sooner of been at home with his family enjoying New Years Eve. A supposed vagrant entered the bar and stood at the counter waiting to be served. The crowd that had gathered at the taps complained amongst themselves that he stunk and shouldn't be served. Oblivious to their comment the man continued to wait, even after everybody had been served. 'What you want, Mate? The barman asked, just a drink please, was the reply - a pint? - Yeah, please. Unsure of where he got his manner, he served him and the man retired to a seat, next to Alan. Alan gasped at the smell of sweat and smoke drenched wet clothes but he was more afraid than anything. He had encountered the plight of insanity before. And homelessness was a symptom.

It was about time I made my way home but there was time yet to have another drink and settled for a pint next door at The George. Here was the local fraternity of elderly decrepit villains and postgraduate students. I took my drink and sat by the door. Tentatively I tried to make conversation with the bloke next to me about what he was reading. 'Fishing quotas, apparently North Sea Cod was in decline and the fishermen of the south were trawling deeper and further away from international waters in an effort to maintain their livelihood. 'Sure, I agreed. Probably in decline like the growth of the population and the price of drugs on the street, who cares no international EU agreement, would stop the Spaniards screwing us out of our share of the cod', we both laughed and he offered me a pint. 'Sure I said I'll always accept a bevy, to which he replied - go get one then....' I recognized the rejection. Many times during my time friends had taken money from me and then told me to buy my own drink. I persevered and apologized for my transgression of speech, explaining why I had come out to the city looking for some security and maybe even something to believe in. Upon laying this depth of emotion on him his defenses and prejudice weakened and soon the conversation although tenuous, turned into an intelligent discourse on the human race.

We spoke about relationships and sex from behind the closet of masculinity. Like talking to a priest at confession. Both of us, and I could conclude all of us had suffered at the hands of love in our search for it. He spoke of his new baby and the stress and late nights and exhaustion it brings. He confessed his love for his wife and their future together, the commitment they had made. He also lamented at the tough course he had taken in university and the boredom of working with statistics for a living. Which to his dismay didn't pay what it was worth and he was often struggling with debt and unemployment as well as family. I tried cheering him up with my own contrasting story of failure to graduate and make a success of my life. The lack of structure and meaning in my life was the bane of all that failed me. 'If only I still had my job down at the cement works, I wouldn't be aimless' or so I thought. Though I knew the meaning of life was the product of a life's work and error, not a nine to five occupation or your time spent in the pub. Though you could be sure it was understood if you could laugh at yourself. I spoke of romance, which amused him a little as I reeled off all the failed love affairs I had had and the effect it had on my growth as a person, blaming a lack of intimacy for my languishing in the mire of unemployment and failure to commit myself to anything other than my next bender. All of which he took with the comical slant I gave it. I thought I had made another friend.

Having concluded our discussion he left to return to his hotel, leaving me behind to consider our meeting. I rolled a smoke and mused on what it was I wanted from life and how I could understand what drove me. I did not know my own capability. Under my own influence I could not change the way I felt about the bigger points of life such as love or my understanding of it. My mind was still chaotic with challenged beliefs and outworn excuses. I suited to distract myself and looked around the bar.

Abbey had been called out to the George late tonight. There had been a disturbance at the bar and as she was the emergency psychiatrist, she had been called to attend the scene. The police were nowhere to be seen as usual, though the local fraternity of doormen had gathered around the entrance waiting for a scene to erupt. A funny one they hoped. Abbey had dressed down for the occasion as she usually did. Looking around the bar nothing seemed the matter, all was well. She approached the bar and asked for information. The barman replied the character had settled and was in the corner by the door with an exchange student. Turning to look, she could see the man talking nonsense to the cornered student who was bemused with his first experience of the city. She adopted a persona and made her advance to help the guy out.

The bar was lively and the miscreants that inhabited its walls were in full spirit doing their own quintessentially neurotic things. An old hippy, that looked like John Lennon sat throwing a spinning beer mat into the air while an old hag plied her trade round each table looking for the deadly desperate and deviant, and a foreign exchange student read a map of the city upside-down in the corner so as not to attract attention. I saw my chance to cause some mischief and crossed the bar to wind him up. I sat and enquired about why he was reading the A-Z. He told me, after a short pause in his broken English, that he had arrived in Liverpool that day to start his studies at the University. He had gotten lost and ended up in Dingle, past Toxteth a rough part of the world indeed and had bought the map to find his way around. That much made sense at least, although I could not be relied upon to make any sense at all, even to a foreigner after a night on the sauce.

My drunken façade as a plastic scouser, soon unnerved him as I began to explain my supposed life history to him as a rock star. I told him I was in a band and had been in several famous ones in my time as a guitarist. In my own mind I was sure of it although in my heart wasn't convinced and my lie was confounded when I made excuses for not being able to play anything he had heard of. I changed my story to save face and instead claimed to know Kurt Cobain, as he was still alive and living on the Wirral. Amused at my wherewithal he bought me a drink.

When he got back from the bar the old hag was at the table offering to score me some rock and show me a good time. I had declined the invitation and tried to send her on her way but she was not leaving me alone that easily whilst the drink was flowing. Seeing I was a weak target she persisted telling me her 'man' was nearby and it would be no trouble to helping me score. The exchange student laughed at my attempts to communicate I wasn't interested but her persistence was scary. I was waiting for the moment to leave them both behind when the doormen ushered her outside to the sound of police radios. The exchange student laughed at me seeing I was not at home here either and raised his glass.

I continued bullshitting the exchange student for another half hour or more before taking my leave later than expected and had missed the train. Knowing I could not hang around the city all night I made my way to the Mersey Tunnel entrance and in a moment or two slipped unseen, inside and towards where I thought there were some fire doors in the side of the wall.

But there wasn't any. I turned back on my heel and faced the entrance to the tunnel, I took a step towards it and then bright lights appeared from the roundabout. Hurtling towards me at 50+ miles per hour I didn't stand a chance. The car swerved and glanced me on my left, screeching to a halt about 30 yards further down the tunnel. I lay motionless on the wet tarmac. I could just about make out the tail lights of the red Proton as I slipped into unconsciousness

DEAD CITY STREETS

The dream ended when I descended some stairs and passed through a strong steel fire door that opened out into the first segment of the tunnel. I turned on the lights and looked around myself. The road surface was above me and the walls of the tunnel curved round to form a half cylinder of concrete with a path about 7 meters across leading downwards on an incline. Lights lit the path from the side drains, to the next door about 100 yards away. All along the walls there were signs prohibiting smoking. I took my first step into the unknown with a little trepidation and fear. There was no telling what I may find on my journey.

Through the fire door and into the second segment I found the same layout as the first. As was the third and fourth and fifth. I traveled quickly through each segment from one end to the other scared out of my wits by the sense of being alone. Should I fall and have an injury here I was unlikely to be found and would surely perish. The hush except for the road above was deafening and the thud of my boots on the shining white path echoed and reverberated from the ceiling to the walls. I looked behind me as I neared the next fire door, I felt like someone was following me, or watching.

For the following few stretches of tunnel I checked them out for cameras or ghosts. I had no idea where this trip would end or whether I would get out the tunnel at all. For about fifteen minutes I paced along through each of the cubicles turning this way and that. I was live on adrenaline. Like an acid trip it made the whole experience of making the journey vivid and exciting. At the end of the next tunnel there was no door in the wall but a corridor taking the path right, up some steps. This could be the end of the road I thought, but no, I was still going downwards. On reaching the top of the stairs realized I had made it to the banks of the Mersey.

As I ascended the steel steps to the top of the tower I wondered what I was discovering. I had no knowledge of the structure of the Mersey tunnels. I had certainly not noticed the towers dominate the skyline opposite each other on the banks of the river. I had no idea what it was I was climbing or where it would lead.

I reached the top of the stairs and opened the fire door into a tall room with three huge circular turbines. The size of them made me stare in wonder. They reached high above me, to the ceiling about one hundred foot up they lay in a state of disrepair, parts having been removed and tools scattered about the place covered in dust. I wondered how long it had been since they had seen human contact. I doubted anyone had been in this room for ten years or more. I rummaged through the clutter and confusion looking for any interesting curios I may like to take home. I climbed some steps to look inside the turbine and found a stack of teen porn sat on a chair. I flicked through a few and took the best copy for myself, stuffing it in my jacket pocket. Looking above me I could climb a ladder to the roof and look out across the estuary from a vantage point two hundred foot above the city. I climbed the ladder and opened the hatch.

DEAD CITY STREETS

Outside on the roof I could see the traffic passing through the city and the flicker of the orange street lamps all across Merseyside and the Wirral. The wind blew a gale up here and I was afraid to get close to the edge, should it blow me off. The Isle of Man ferry was lit up in all it's splendor by the lights of the Liver Buildings and I could hear the roar of the wind and feel the cold of the river. The air smelt of spent fuel and salt. Looking around me I could see for miles, even as far as the lights of the Welsh hills and Lancashire, behind. In an instant I was caught in a panic of the height I was at I quickly made my way back to the hatch and descended the ladder, clouting my head on the lid as I closed the hatch and nearly falling the twenty foot down the ladders. Still in a panic, I made my way back down the route I had climbed to the tower, back to the tunnel.

Outside of the fire doors I could hear traffic passing through to its destination. I opened the opposite door to that I had just come from and entered the passage. In the safety of the evacuation tunnel and it luminescence I took a rest. I had been walking for what seemed like hours and still saw no end to the adventure, as it was turning out to be. I rolled a smoke and lit it. Taking care not to cause any fires I enjoyed inhaling the confidence building cancer stick as a gust of wind ripped through the tunnel walls. Rolling it on my tongue and taking my time I was sure of getting out of here. And was soon on my feet again and ready to move on.

The following stretch of path meandered under the

rush of late night traffic for ever. Deviating this way and that and forever downwards the shape of the cylinders began to change and the roof got lower at the entrances and exits as I passed through countless sections of the construction. I thought I was alone down here. Out of sight and silent. But I got an eerie feeling as I walked that something knew I was down here. I could hear the trickling sound of water running in the gutter to the right, coming from the road above. How on earth it reached the river confused me, until I saw a manhole cover bedded into the floor of the path ahead.

A feeling came over me much like a dream you have when you have not slept for days. I could see in my minds eye a whole new exotic, beautiful and dangerous world underneath the lid of the drain. Warm with fresh breezes but always night wherever. I could see a tall man talking to his only friend while a child skipped about the meadows in the dark, whilst all the time I sat and despaired at my fate to be unloved.

As I trod on the cover I felt someone or something was following and I upped my pace to escape the feeling of being perused. When I looked behind I thought I could feel two ghostly hands reach up out of the pit and grab for my legs. In the distance I could hear the sound of footsteps and fire doors slamming behind me. I ran, as quickly as I could from the threat to the end of the tunnel and through the door. And the next one and the next one and the next one, I didn't count how many until I reached a dead end. A sheer concrete wall faced me. I waited for a moment to see if the footsteps caught up, but they stopped. I had no choice but to turn on my pursuer and face whatever was following. I paced back to a door I had passed several sections back, but there was no sign of anyone. Relieved, I set about searching for a way out. I managed to open the door I had passed and into a corridor.

Through the corridor was a flight of concrete steps and I entered another corridor made of brick walls either side with gaps in the construction. Along it ran a pipe and across it sat a tractor raised above the floor on stilt like legs. It looked like a huge predatory spider, its lights staring at me through the black soot of the air. I hesitated making my progress to be sure it didn't move. Then in an anxious state hurried alongside the pipeline and into the dark, I moved swiftly thinking the spider would come to life and devour me. I even thought I saw its shadow scuttle down the cylinder after me as I reached the end of the path.

Through the gaps in the wall were pieces of engineering equipment and twelve foot boards of plywood covered in dust. Every so often was a door hidden behind a roughly constructed wall, I ignored the first few and decided to follow the cave to the end and find an exit there. I wondered what this place was for. Sure a pipeline ran through it, possibly laid there by the spider but the whole oblong room was eerie and wicked. Somehow in the pitch black several thousand feet underground,

I could see without any light. It was as if light had been captured within the corridor many generations ago and stayed there. The place was covered in dust and littered with cardboard boxes. As I neared the end of the path I saw a red door ahead of me. I opened the door and escaped the nightmare.

Through the door was a turn in the path. It lead me upwards in a spiral to a higher cylindrical tunnel and then a straight length of path looking much like a spaceship corridor, lit on both sides. I followed it to the end and then leading upwards to a chasm in the wall. I stopped knowing the danger I was in, should I take this path I would surely end up dead. That much was certain. In front of me a stream of fresh water flowed into the chasm of the queer shaped construction. I jumped over it and landed half in it soaking myself up to the knees. I shimmied to the top of the incline and looked into the chasm. I could see now this was the underground rail network I had reached. I could go no further. I had no choice but to turn back and face my fears again. I made a cigarette and turned to go. Under the flow of the river I faced the spider that inhabited it again.

Back through the spiders web I thought I could see lights ahead of me. I stopped and hid behind the cover of wall, waiting for them to come towards me but they faded into the dark. Upon trying to open the door out, I found that the exit was locked from the other side and I could not get out. I contemplated my predicament. Should I get stuck here I would never be found alive and up until this minute I had no idea of what direction I was traveling in, let alone if I could find my way out. I had faith in myself enough though, to believe I would. I said a silent prayer to God, any God that would secure my passage out of the spaceship I seemed to be a part of right now, '...I forgive you everything, my Lord – but the world can go to hell.' I looked to the spider to check it had not moved and set off back into the dark of the bricked up walls and dust looking for another exit.

I tried one of the doors further down the corridor, tucked behind a wall. Reaching through into the darkness I could not see a thing. I daren't step into such blackness. Like a void nothing was beneath my feet. I took a step back and returned to the spider's door. Another prayer, 'Ok Lord please give me the strength to open this door and I forgive you and the earth my whole life and everything in it.' Looking around I found a crowbar left at the foot of the steps and used it to try and force the door open. It did. I believed for that moment I had reached Jesus for once in my life. I was grateful for the blessing I had received. Checking out the situation I believed my anxiety had gotten the better of me and there was nothing to fear. I stepped back into the mire. Back in the corridor I checked another door to see if I could continue the journey.

Behind it, the rush of early morning traffic took its passengers to there destination on the banks. I looked out across the road. On the far side was another evacuation tunnel. I had one chance to get out of here. Checking no vehicles where in sight I pushed through the door and raced across the road surface to the other side. Hopping onto the ledge and into the doorway I had made it.

I didn't stick around. Soon the police would be on the scene and I knew I must keep moving. Sure enough as I hastened through the dim light of the evacuation shaft I heard the sound of sirens and the slowing of traffic behind. In blind panic I ran from my pursuers up the slight gradient of the path towards the still far distant hope of tomorrow morning greeting me on the banks of Seacombe.

I moseyed along for what felt like hours. Having evaded capture and conquered my fears of the unknown I was on a high that drugs don't do. I had the clarity of mind that could have cut wool with my teeth. Everything that had been of concern to me was rounding up and making sense like never before. Even my sense of being without a partner was put into perspective, after all their where potential love interests about for my delectation all I had to do was commit myself in spirit and pocket to their needs and make a union. It was all a bit mushy for me though. I wanted something with a bit more spice. Not the traditional love at first sight and marriage but someone who could share my emotional depth and wonder. I had one friend in particular in mind.

Up some more steps I discovered a bunker, deep underground where the Mersey tunnel staff took their coffee breaks. Looking around all seemed quiet. I settled down to rest my legs and help myself to a cuppa. A camera on the wall facing me recorded my movements. I didn't care, I was home and dry. I read yesterdays paper and put my feet up on the chairs. Enjoying the calm of the room I ignored the knock that came from the next room - what I assumed to be the machine room. I waited several minutes before checking the door. I could see that it had been locked from the other side and whoever was behind had been spooked by my arrival. I returned to my seat and had another cuppa with the last of the milk and flicked through some porn magazines left under the sink. I wanted to sleep but still had to travel maybe ten miles, by foot home. As eight o'clock struck, I emptied my cup in the sink and went back into the labyrinth of tunnels, looking for an unseen exit.

I found it, a ladder reaching up above to the tunnel entrance at Queensway on the banks of Merseyside. The daylight hurt my eyes as I pushed at the lid that covered the shaft. Then closing the lid behind me I made a start out of the gaping hole in the earth that had been my search for new ground to resolve past fears. People passing in their cars could not believe their eyes as I raced out into the morning sun, hoping the police would not pick me up for trespass. A car stopped at the ticket booth and the occupant asked what I was doing under the tunnel. 'Arming a nuclear arsenal, I replied. He shit himself…

The roads that led home deviated this way and that. I took to the back streets through the towns and villages, away from the by – pass, to escape the stare of commuters in passing cars. Still the everyday folk in the town centers would give me a second look as I made my way. Exhausted I stopped at a back - street church of sorts, a Lutheran chapel. Moving some chairs aside I settled on the floor and made myself comfortable for the first time in days, I drifted off.

I don't know where I woke. I wasn't in hospital and had no recollection of the accident in the tunnel. The room had a small bench on which I was laid out with a thin cotton cloth spread over it. I looked around and finding the scene inexplicable sat looking down at the carpet – tiled floor wondering where on earth I had gotten to. Suddenly I heard the sound of the chapel door closing.

Two people sat on the chairs in front of me, paying their respects to Jesus in silence. I lay there for a moment, then set to my feet and made for the door. It was locked. I asked the two worshippers where I might find a way out. They waited a few seconds before telling me, I almost believed I was invisible, dead even, 'Ask him,' was the reply. Flummoxed for a moment, I sat with them in silent contemplation of the crucifixion scene on the wall. Spirituality was a prevalent theme in my life but never had I gave my faith to the Christian church. I waited for a revelation, a sign, a wonder. None came. I laughed out loud.

I finally knew who I was. It felt strange.

I heard a key turn in the door and I made for the exit. The vicar opened the door and let me out with

DEAD CITY STREETS

a nod of his head and a shake of it too. Once outside again I started headlong along Chester Road and into Bebington. Past the stores and streets of the old village I arrived in the wooded park of the Mersey Ferry, in Eastham. Here I rested again, on a park bench. Pulling my coat off and laying it over me I tried to sleep but soon the cold and rain of the estuary blew through the forest and woke me to the sound of approaching voices. Immediately I recognized them as teenagers, Chavs. They approached, and took interest in the sight of a young vagrant down on his luck. I huddled under the coat listening to their conversation. The tallest one gave me a prod; I pulled back the coat and looked into his eyes. 'He's alright, he called to his friends who stood a distance away. 'Is he dead? Asked one of the girls, No' he replied. I sat upright and rubbed the sleep from my eyes. 'Are you alright, mate? The tallest asked. 'Yeah I said, jus' getting' away for a bit. 'OK, he said and went to join his friends. I sat in the cool mist watching them move away into the forest and made a pipe.

The lighter I had was nearly out of gas and I struggled to take a drag on the hot smoke, burning my fingers but not the dope. I gave up and chose to leave this place and take a walk around the grounds of the forest. As I entered the clearing I was surprised to see one of my brothers tending to a Shire horse. I went over and asked him why he was there. Apparently their was a family fete going on in the park, involving traditional crafts such as charcoal burning and wood turning and his own reason for being there, 'working' horses. I attempted to make conversation hoping for some sympathy but he was too busy for my bother and told me that I could not stay while he was working. Knowing I had just been told to lose myself, I waved him goodbye and went back into the forest in the direction of the lane that would take me home.

Once back on the road I slowed down the pace. I had traveled about fifteen miles in a single morning through every town and village on the southerly bank of the Mersey. I took a short cut down the dock road that ran alongside the ship canal and into my home town. Other than a lorry that passed alongside me as I walked I saw no other signs of life. A great orange oil tanker passed upstream on the canal, sounding its horn as it passed. The waves lapped the walls of the embankment that I walked on and stirred behind in it's wake. Here I took to the rail tracks that would lead me to the industrial estate behind the street I lived on. I jumped between each sleeper, tripping and slipping as I did. Each was greater than my gait and this slowed my progress more. The walk became a leisurely stroll in the tundra, enjoying the sunshine that broke through the clouds and taking deep breaths of the sweet damp air. As I made it to the industrial estate behind my home the traffic became busier and wagons hauled their cargos along the narrow supply roads between factories.

Across the rail bridge, where I had discarded my cannabis years previously, and onto the streets of

DEAD CITY STREETS

home, I had made it back to a place of safety. I put my key in the door to enter the family home with no knowledge of what was waiting there for me. It was locked, with a deadlock or so it seemed as the key wouldn't turn. I went round the back through the alley between the terraces to see if the back door was open. No luck there either. To my right though I could see the lounge window was open. I reached inside to clip the runners opened it wide and crawled through the windowpane.

The house was quiet. I looked round each of the rooms for my family, none were home. Settling in front of the TV, I could see something was amiss. The house had changed somehow though I could not put my finger on it. I ignored the flash of recognition and changed channels looking for some light entertainment. Nothing was on. I searched for my mother's cigarettes down the side of the chair and found 40 Marlboro, not her usual brand – on the fireplace. Lighting one up I went to the kitchen for something to eat. Searching through the cupboards, there was plenty of fresh food but nothing I really wanted to eat. Seeing my mother had left a cooked meal in the microwave for my sister, I set the microwave to full power and helped myself to a large vodka from the Smirnoff bottle, in the fridge.

Thinking I was home alone I decided to have a look at some porn and so went up to my room to fetch my magazines. The room had changed. The bed and carpet were the same but the room was filled with other pieces of furniture that I didn't recognize.

A couch and computer desk. I assumed mother was having a change around. Maybe she was going to make things up with me?

Looking under the bed, I found a magazine that wasn't my own but with much cuter models. I laughed out loud at the thought of my father or someone leaving such a gift for me and immediately set about jerking the gerkin. As I did I could hear some movement in the room next to me. I quickly shut the door thinking it was the dog or I had failed to realize my sister was home and continued. Well it had never bothered anyone any other time had it? I was just reaching the point of no return when the door flung open and stood in the doorway was a small child of about 5. 'Oi, you little slag! I shouted, and jumped up and closed the door with my appendage still hanging out my flies. First I thought my youngest sister was playing up and after cleaning myself up I went to the next room, my brothers' to find her.

She was hiding under the bed. I told her to not do that again and went back downstairs, shrugging off the embarrassment. Strangely something seemed different about her at that moment. Her hair was darker. She was cuter and she seemed more afraid of me. I ignored my worries and thought I would deal with the fallout between myself and my feminine family members later. Something still bugged me though. It was like I had been missing for years and returned to find my family had changed persona's, like in Flight of the Navigator.

DEAD CITY STREETS

Back in front of the TV, I began to relax sipping my drink in large gulps and chain smoking my mother's ciggies. I would get her them back later. Soon I had another vodka and ate my sisters dinner then set up in front of the TV to watch the afternoon news. Stories of terror and hate were being broadcast across the airwaves and absorbed into my mind. I responded to the prompts of the newscaster as they spoke, giving my own opinions on the global terror suspects, war in Iraq and internet pedophiles. Suddenly, I caught a glimpse someone pop their head around the door into the living room. 'Mums' not here John, she said. I waited a few moments then followed her upstairs. I tapped at the door to my sisters room, 'Nardia, where is she? I asked from behind the door. No-one answered. I tried the door but it was locked. 'Nardia, are you in there? - 'No, she's not' was the answer but not my sister's voice. 'Who's that then?' Again there was no answer. A younger voice called for me to 'go away.' I shrugged my shoulders, shook my head in confusion, and turned to go back downstairs. Behind the door I could hear the strange girl making a call. 'Someone's here! I heard her say.

Back downstairs I helped myself to another extra large Smirnoff and continued to smoke, breaking into a fresh packet of 20 Marlboro from beside the couch...I switched on the light, found a scrap of paper and set about writing a short poem about my state of mind.

As I wrote, some commotion began to erupt outside. I could see one of my neighbors in the street, staring in through the net curtains, holding a beer can and laughing right at me. I ignored him and continued to scribble away at the page. Soon he was back with a friend; both stared in through the window smiling at me and raised their cans of beer in a salute. 'Knobheads.., I thought and continued to try and get my ideas down on paper. Then the door went. *At last*, I thought, Mums home! I waited for her to come in and start screaming at me to clear off. Instead I heard the voice of a man. Not one I recognized. I could hear the strange girl from upstairs telling the man that 'someone was here' and sounding in quite a panic. The door opened and the face of the voice peered at me from across the room and then closed the door behind him. It was then I noticed the fish tank in the corner, I had not seen it before. Looking around myself I could recognize that some of the features of the room had changed since I last left to go hike. The only thing that hadn't changed of course was the couch and carpet and the dining table that had hidden the fish tank. I realized then I may be in trouble.

An angry face peered round the open door. 'You better leave mate,' was the words, I had no idea what I had walked into. I got to my feet and went to ask the figure who they were and what they were doing in my home, but they hastened out the door leaving me standing alone in the hall to work out the plot. I walked back into the living room asking myself what on earth was going on. Outside a crowd had now gathered. All neighbors from the street. Something was going on outside.

DEAD CITY STREETS

Suspecting a bomb scare I ventured outside to find out what was going on.

From the doorstep, I could see a scene had erupted in the street. Police cars parked both sides of the road and my neighbors and friends being pushed back from the kerb. A friend across the street called out for me to 'get out of here!' 'What's goin' on? I shouted back, all around there was laughter. 'Jesus, get out! He said. I stepped back inside to collect my coat, again there was laughter. I made my exit.

On stepping out the door to join the crowd I could see two plain clothes policemen hid behind the cover of their car. First I walked to Paul, to ask where the bomb was. He roared with laughter and walked off down his garden path shaking his head. Even more perplexed by now with the afternoon's events, I went in the opposite direction across the road and on to the intended destination of Sim's to find out. As I crossed, one of the policemen raced up behind me and, I thought hit me in the back. At once I felt nauseated and I had a sudden pain in my chest. I was keeling over and had to sit down with my back to the garden fence. The CID officer approached and said just this, 'you're nicked, mate! Without pausing to let me recover from my seizure, he and another copper bundled me into the back of the panda and set off for the next town's constabulary.

Chapter 5

London Gig

I felt like a VIP on the way to my destination choosing any cabin or seat I liked. When I first boarded the intercity link however, I had no idea where I was going or why. Though the reason I had came to be at this station platform in the early hours of the morning was the age old one. I had left the police station in Chester in the middle of the night having not been charged with anything, to hang out at the station looking for someone to talk to. I had not eaten and had not spoken to anyone who had any sense in weeks. While I smoked on the benches the last of the late night commuters raced homeward to enjoy new years day. I would not be having one. As the station closed for the night I chose to hide in the shadows so I would not be seen by the staff. When I saw my chance I hopped aboard an intercity express train to keep warm. I had no idea that it would be leaving shortly. When it did I was glad to be leaving this stinking city to find new horizons. And just maybe I could find someone to talk to.

The train traveled non-stop through the countryside of Cheshire and the Midlands at speed. I sat looking out the window, smoking and drinking some cheap super strength cider. It felt good to be on the move away from what I had known. I hoped something substantial would result from my venture into the unknown. I did not want to spend this New Year alone. As the train raced towards its destination I took on the issues life had given me to work through. The problems I had would not go away by ignoring them; I had to make my peace with the world and its neighbor. This new year I had the chance of new life if I could just settle my grievances.

I had reached the Birmingham terminus at about 1.20am.Having travelled all this way I had little inclination to stay here it would be cold outside I had brought nothing to eat. This running away from home business was roughing it all right. I didn't't want to go home until I had sorted my emotional situation. So it was in my interest to try and travel further, but the opportunity wasn't to be forthcoming.

Lifting myself out of my seat I found my way to some stairs that would take me up to the main corridor to the main foyer of the station. Taking each step with some thought I reached the kiosks and ticket counter. I looked around. In this huge hall there were few people about only some railway engineers and a young couple standing by the entrance. I considered asking them for help to stay alive here, after all I would need it, but chose to play it safe and give away my intentions to no-one, that way I could secure my own safety.

Reaching into my pocket I took out some change. I had the good fortune to have a few pounds to my name and chose to invest a pound in a hot cup of coffee at the coffee bar there. I ordered my drink and sat down. I stared out into the hall surrounding me taking in the movements of the five people there with me, when a well dressed youngster carrying a satchel strolled into the station. The holy man had arrived. I watched his movements and those of the others. The young couple where petting each other in the corner near the doors. The engineers clambered about the scaffold lifting the false ceiling. The holy man approached me.

He sat down and faced me. He was well dressed boy of about 20 and wore traditionally patterned but modern clothes his hat was that of a Rastafarian, or Sikh. Introducing himself as Schlingeer he asked where I was going. A normal question you might think but in my crazed mind it was a rhetorical question. I replied that I had no idea where I was heading to, which is true I didn't't. We sat in stony silence for a few minutes not knowing why we were sat at the same table. Then I began to talk.

I asked him about the things that concerned me. I told him about my problems and that I had made myself intentionally homeless.   He seemed concerned at this not for my safety but for his own. This made me laugh. I decided to ask him if he felt safe to which he didn't reply. I began to talk religion.

It had been a long time before I had read anything on religion, but still asked him about his faith. He was reluctant to give away any of the details of his beliefs which I expected but unfortunately due to my state of mind I told him some of mine which would of have been a pretty stupid thing to do

DEAD CITY STREETS

considering I was in a foreign town and what had been occupying my mind but it was obvious to all that met with me that I was clearly mad.

I was unperturbed by this but as I talked he became increasingly more worried - looking as I explained how I had come to be here in Birmingham. I told him of my flight from my home town in the middle of the night my awakening to my dark side, my experience of death, comfort and family. I told him all that bothered me, including my search to be loved. It comes as no surprise that he was shocked and confused that I would want to share all this with a stranger. I told him it helped.

As our talk went on I began to equate my situation with that of my friends and brothers. Would they of ran away from home in the middle of the night to pursue a life on the streets. I thought not. Why had I? I recalled the events of the past week. The attitude of my friends towards me, the entrenched position of my mother on my living arrangements and my depth of pity, due to my single status all raced through my mind with such weight that I could of struck him. Which was a shame, seeing as he was the only good company I had met with in a week or more?

The coffee shop was closing for the night now and the assistant moved us on from our seats. The guy must have thought that he had been saved by the bell and moved on ahead of me to the doors and struck up conversation with the couple. I stood by a route map and studied its direction. London was just a train ride south. I moved on over to the ticket counter and queried the clerk on how much it cost to get to London. It was more than I had. I let out a cuss and asked how far the fifteen pounds I had in my pocket would get me. Not far came the reply. I was stuck here for the duration or until morning at least. I chose to take a stride outside.

As I passed through the line of doors next to the young couple I looked at the pair of them in the eyes. They both seemed very much in love, why they should come to be with me in this place, at this time was a mystery. The tall black man of the couple raised his hand as he passed through the doors. I was outside.

In the dim light of the taxi rank, I took in the senses of the city. The smell, sound, taste, sights the ambience. In the distance and all around me was the ever present rumble of distant traffic and air conditioning systems. A bus pulled away from its stop, spewing gases into the air and making me cough. It was deserted. Nothing stirred here in the inner city. Nothing except a cool breeze and the trickle of yesterdays drizzle in the gutter.

I walked to the left in an effort to walk round the terminus. If I could find my way round then I could find somewhere to doss for the night. It was cold out here and I wasn't prepared to be spending lots of time outdoors. I had to find shelter. I walked slowly taking in my direction so I could find my way back. There was nothing but deserted street after street. I stopped and sat to make a cigarette on some steps and looked around. I had come all this way and for what, I thought. To catch pneumonia and die? I was soaked through and cold. My back had begun to ache like I was exhausted as well. I smoked my cigarette and rose to my feet again.

Across the other side of the street was a public toilet. I took a look to see if I could find some rest here but it was closed. On the other side of the road though there was a multi story car park. Inside the lift tower it was dry enough to bed down. I took a chance to stay here for a few hours. My back by now was really sore and as I struggled to choke back the catarrh on my throat I rubbed my back to put some heat into it. Using my bag as a pillow I lay down to rest.

The early morning had been both clammy and damp. I had not slept. The early morning brought no relief from the elements and I was in agony. My back has caught cold during the night on the floor and ached worse than the day before. Rising to my feet, I nearly passed out. I could barely stay conscious in this much pain. I lifted the back of my sweater to look at the area. My left lower back was red and had become swollen and red. I must have dragged myself all the way to the public cubicle across the road cussing and swearing not knowing how close to the edge I was. I washed my face and took another look at my back. It seemed fine other than the swelling but it was sore as having a red hot poker drawn into your back.

Back outside in the deserted streets I wandered as

far as I could without getting lost, always listening for some sound of life. Passing one open window two stories above a bar I could her 'someone' having furious sex, with themselves it would seem. It amused me that someone suffered the same fate as me here. Nearby, the street cleaning cart raced about the place cleaning an already immaculate street. I had forgotten what time of year it was during my trip. I just wanted to get away from home so I wouldn't be alone.

Still losing consciousness, I dragged myself to the terminus nearly passing out with each step. The construction workers outside the station stared at me. Being a bank holiday the station was still at a standstill at five in the morning. It was time I contacted my mother. I put my change in the phone and got the number off my mobile. It rang. She answered from her pillow. She was not happy to hear from me at this hour of the morning. I explained to her how I had come to be in a far away town in the midlands, the midlands? No, after telling her the name of the station it appeared I was in London! Before ringing off she told me to make my own way home. My concern now was how I was to get home on New Years Day... She had made clear to me that she wouldn't be able to help me get home today. Again I was on my own in a strange town with no way home.

I sat on the floor in the middle of the hall by a 'tie rack' and struggled to consider my options through the agony of my abdominal pain. I could be here for days until the New Year was over. I would need to find some information to secure my passage home. But I was too weak to lift myself of the floor. Summoning superhuman strength I gathered myself to my feet, just in time to see the holy man return.

He stood next to me and grunted a hello. I wondered where he spent the night.

I managed to raise my hand to acknowledge him. He seemed worried about something; I could recognize the fear on his face. 'What's the matter' is what I asked. His lips moved in a whisper but I didn't understand what it is he said. I did hear the word 'sorry…. Kim.' He probably asked me the same question. I was weak and feverish I asked him if he had any painkillers. In a moment he was gone and back again with some pills. I swallowed these without water and took my place on the benches. The holy man came with me.

It was at this point I realized I had an injury. My back was getting more painful by the minute. I looked for the tell tale smear of blood. Immediately I thought I understood how I had gained the injury I wanted to get home and quick. I was losing consciousness and was talking incoherently. I told Schlingeer I may possibly die and he considered his position. He went to the ticket desk to enquire whether any trains left today. One, my one did.

On returning the holy man ushered me to the platform I had come from, just as the tannoy announced the next train to Crewe was ready to leave. We took the stairs down to the waiting room where it was warm. Upon sitting down I nearly fell asleep, but the holy man would not let me miss my train and forever wonder what happened to me. When the slide doors opened he helped me onto the carriage and we said our goodbyes. He was glad to see me gone. The doors closed and I was on my way.

The return home was comfortable. My back became numb and I was alert to the towns we passed through. I made a joint and smoked it openly. With no one else on the train I didn't't have to worry about being caught. As the journey passed I considered my experience. In all my life I had not felt so down as I did this New Year. It was evident I had reached the end of my tether. I could not go on like this. The holy man had opened my eyes to the suffering I had put myself through in an effort to find security and love. He represented the success that had recently eluded me. The promise of better times ahead. This New Year was to bring new life for those like me.

I arrived back home at my fathers at around six in the morning. The sky was like dusk and the black clouds of night rolled away with a silver of light in the west while the half moon still hung way up in the east. The bird twittered on the roof tops and the pigeons called to they're mate. I raced through town with my hood covering my head. Upon reaching my father's, I knocked and waited for an answer while he fumbled for keys. After a few moments he answered and allowed me in.

DEAD CITY STREETS

'Where you been, he asked me.

'London' I said.

'Oh.' Is all he said and set about making toast.

'What do you know?'

'Well, I said, nothing really - I got lost.'

I sat in the chair opposite the window for maybe an hour biting my lip. I hated all I knew. There was no trust between me and my brothers or mother, my friends followed there own agenda. I was out of breath. I tried my father for answers.

'Why... I said, is everyone against me? What have I done wrong?' he didn't have an answer. He just sat eating his toast.

'Well, he said, I don't know. Have you done anything wrong?

I had been asking myself the same question. I didn't know either.

'Do you know where your mother is now? My father asked.

'No, was my answer. The previous few days where still a blur to me. I was confused and aggravated by my experience, frightened and uncomfortable too. I had one clue to go on. But I was scared of holding a dear dream high in my mind, 'should it upset someone.

My father asked again.

'Well there's just one thing, I said, there's this girl.'

My father nearly choked on his toast. Arrrgg! He stood up and put his plate in the sink. I could hear him washing his plate but not what he said. Meanwhile the voices teased me under my breath as I wrapped my arms around myself and tried to shed a tear.

DEAD CITY STREETS

Chapter 6

Hospital Beds

A day later, I was admitted to hospital under a section 2. Detained for assessment that is. I arrived at the front gate at 6 pm and was quickly ushered inside. I sat in the dining hall waiting to see a nurse quite aware of my situation. I had to admit something was wrong. I had been consumed with hate and fear for all I knew. I didn't realize that the changes I had been going through were to blame.

I was served pea soup with cold curry and rice. It was the first thing I had eaten in over a week and in spite of its lack of culinary delight, I enjoyed its nourishment and felt better immediately. I was over the worst of the nightmare. Soon I was taken to the doctor's study and given my assessment by a woman who was the identical twin of my mother. Basic questions about my beliefs, fears and family were asked of me. I felt no more hate. I told the nurse that. I was happy to stay.

The assessment over, I was led to a single room with a bed a blanket and a cupboard, nothing more. Lying on the bed staring at the ceiling I could still hear the sound of passing cars on the road. White noise. The ghosts that haunted me had gone for the time being. The taunts and insults had gone away. The one thing my conscience had to say to me was I was sorry. An empty mind was presented to me. I settled under the bed sheets and drifted off into a sweet dream.

Chapter 7

Recovery

So, what can I say about my breakdown and 8 years therapy? The most important thing I feel I must say is Schizophrenia is no mystery. As my Doctor said after I was admitted to hospital for the 3rd time, 'Drugs take their toll.'

It's true, but I have to differ on some of the triggers of the symptoms of the illness.

My breakdown, I believe was a result of those early choices I made to smoke cannabis and do other drugs, and that was the lifestyle I lived - true.

However, the real story is that when I decided to change at 20, the past lives of others in my life defeated the new path I wanted to follow... The friends I had back then assumed I would always be there for them. That is the start of the story you have just read. Take a look at the beginning now... because this is what I was running from.

What I am trying to say is this; the negativity around me during this time was the trigger for the madness. The voices themselves, (should you understand what I mean) are a long drawn out thought process that considers the present influences, and often tell you of the negativity being left at your doorstep, as my astrologer says, 'Like a baby Moses.' But a lot of this single minded speaking out loud has to do with the shit they put into cannabis these days. But that's not the complete picture.

Those old friends from my past didn't want me leaving them behind and I was not sure I could survive on my own. So eventually the negativity of the druggie lifestyle I was living with my old friends, caught me up and took control of my life when I really wanted to get away and lead my new life with my then, girlfriend.

I am sorry to say, it did not work out. My girlfriend and I split, and I dealt with it by getting off it. So this is no love story.

I made a deal with myself after this final stay in hospital to give up my addictions and settle for some other kind of life. One that is more stable and secure. That is the life I lead now. I smoke less than I have ever done and intend to give up completely and have another stab at life. You know, the car, kids and house, instead of some coke den. It can only be positive. And it's taken 8 years to get this far. I honestly think I can make it, this time.

I remember asking my doctor and nurse who assessed me, if schizophrenia was permanent. I can conclude if you continue popping pills and coke and speed and weed down your neck for a certain period of time then yes, you're fucked. And what's more, as I am sure you know, the shit sticks!

This is my own take on madness. I don't expect anyone else's to be the same and neither should you. Having been in hospital, I know we each had our own problems to deal with, and the healthcare professionals will do their best by each of us.

To finish up, I know better now. Have a career or develop a talent, go to college and get a degree, anything is better than the life I have just lived. I am sure of that.

Printed in the United Kingdom by
Lightning Source UK Ltd., Milton Keynes
141394UK00001B/38/P